DISCARD

D0699777

The Evolution and Eradication of Infectious Diseases

Charcot

"Disease is very old and nothing about it has changed. It is we who change as we learn to recognize what was formerly imperceptible."

From an Editorial,
J.A.M.A., 1962, *179:* 800.

Cockburn

Infectious disease is composed of three variables, the host, the pathogen, and the environment. It is in a constant state of flux, capable of changing in step with any variation in any one of its components. New diseases appear, old ones alter, and some may disappear completely.

The Evolution
and Eradication
of
Infectious Diseases

AIDAN COCKBURN, M.D.

THE JOHNS HOPKINS PRESS   BALTIMORE AND LONDON

Copyright © 1963 by The Johns Hopkins Press
All rights reserved
Manufactured in the United States of America

The Johns Hopkins Press, Baltimore, Maryland 21218
The Johns Hopkins Press Ltd., London

ISBN-0-8018-0131-1

Originally published, 1963
Second printing, 1970

Eve, my wife, is to a large degree responsible for this book. Not only did she rewrite much of the original book in 1953, translating my cumbersome and incoherent jargon into good English, but over the years has endeavored to teach me how to express my thoughts in simple language. She has typed out the manuscript at least six times.

But more than this, she has provided many of the ideas. For example, knowing my thoughts on the origin of the treponemes, she recognized the significance of the sketch by Dürer (Plate 9) while visiting an art exhibit in New York.

She has accompanied me on my travels from the snows of northern Alberta to the heat of the tropics and many places in between. In the course of these travels she has reared and educated our five children.

This book is therefore dedicated to my wife, Eve Gillian Cockburn.

Preface and Acknowledgments

THIS IS THE Age of Specialization. The pace of scientific discovery is now so rapid and the mass of collected facts so colossal that no longer can any one man repeat the feat of Leonardo da Vinci and encompass within himself all contemporary learning. It is indeed task enough for the individual specialist merely to keep abreast with the developments in his own narrow field without expecting to be fully informed of any others. Yet, concentration on the particular in this fashion is apt to result in an inability to visualize the general, a situation summed up in the old saying about not being able to see the wood for the trees. This, then, is the justification for the work presented here, which is an attempt to give a birdseye view of the field of the relationships between host, parasite, and environment with particular reference to human infectious disease. It is offered in all humility, with the full knowledge that a specialist in any one of the fifty odd disciplines to which reference is made is likely to find errors and omissions within his special knowledge. In fact, the task is too big for one person: the success of this work is to be measured by the extent to which it stimulates other workers to correct and complete it.

THE OUTLINE of this book was first put on paper in 1953 in a tavern just south of Greeley, Colorado. Dr. Jiri Nehnevajsa, Assistant Professor of Sociology at the University of Colorado, requested me to read a paper at the Conference on World Affairs at his University. He wanted something big, and none of my suggested topics seemed of the required dimensions until, at the end of three hours of somewhat hilarious discussion, we settled on the title of "Infectious Diseases since the Ice Age." Although this paper was never prepared, the summary was submitted to the Communicable Disease Center in Atlanta, Georgia, and approval obtained to make the presentation. Some months later my position with the Communicable Disease Center terminated, but my salary was continued for six months, during which time facilities were provided for me to collect data for a monograph on the lines of the summary. A first draft was completed in Greeley by December 1953.

Ideas on evolution in infectious diseases had been gaining shape in my mind for many years. The earliest seed appeared while I was working in 1937 at the North Eastern Fever Hospital, London County Council, England, and I am indebted to the staff of that hospital for giving me my first intensive instructions on infectious diseases. The ideas on evolution grew during the air-raids of London in 1940–41 when great epidemics were anticipated but did not appear, and in the British Army in the Aldershot Command in 1941–42. My first and most loyal collaborator was Captain Marjery Feachem, Royal Army Medical Corps, in Aldershot, England 1941–42.

Up to this time, my experience had been confined to specifically human infections: It was while serving in the British Army in West Africa, 1942–44, that the role of animal life in human infections struck me most forcibly. In the rain forests and orchard bush of the Gold Coast (Ghana), most infections are influenced by the surrounding animal and plant life to a degree never seen in urban England. At this period I was greatly encouraged and stimulated by the late Brigadier General G. M. Findlay to study the relationship between animal and human infections.

As Hygiene Officer in the British Army in Palestine and Transjordan in 1945–46, I learned much about plague, relapsing fever, typhus, malaria, and entomology from the scientists of that area, particularly the late Professor Mer of Rosh Pinna and Dr. Shulov, Zoologist. To various officers of the Arab Legion I am indebted for an opportunity for studying wild life in some of the more inaccessible regions of their territory.

In Kumasi, Ashanti, I had formed a small zoo and collected bird specimens and parasites, and this led me to the Regents Park Menagerie in London. In 1946–47, as Assistant Superintendent of the Zoological Society of London, I was exposed to the steady and stimulating flow of first class zoologists from all parts of the world, and daily would have the benefit of a dozen or more expert consultations on matters ranging from the ocular fundus of the giraffe, the parasites of the giant panda and okapi, the urino-genitary tract of the wallaby, to the fat content of tigers' urine. In particular, I owe much to Dr. G. M. Vevers, Superintendent of the Society; the late Professor Frederick Wood Jones, Royal College of Surgeons; the late Dr. C. M. Wenyon and Dr. Cecil A. Hoare of the Welcome Research Foundation; the staffs of the British Museum (Natural History) and the London School of Tropical Medicine. In 1947, papers on the evolution of malaria and filaria were written, but these were premature and fortunately were rejected by the editors of the journals to which they were submitted. I am grateful to these editors.

In Canada in 1947–48, Professor William Rowan, University of Alberta, introduced me to the cyclic phenomena of certain animal populations. The late Dr. A. E. Archer and Dr. M. A. R. Young of Lamont Clinic, Alberta, made it possible for me to study for a month the wild life of Elk Island National Park.

In 1948, an invitation to work on the arthropod-borne encephalitis viruses was received from the United States Public Health Service through the interest of Dr. Justin M. Andrews, and for the next five and a half years, I obtained many ideas through contact with the staff of the Communicable Disease Center, Atlanta. Dr. Andrews has been a constant advisor and source of information. As mentioned above, in 1953, the Communicable Disease Center permitted me to spend six months in research on the evolution of infectious diseases, and the main outlines of Chapter 4 were written during this period. The late Dr. Charles R. Rein of New York contributed much to the section on the treponematoses.

I am deeply grateful to the physicians of Ceylon and East Pakistan for teaching me much of what I know of the infections of their areas during my visit 1956–60, especially Dr. Herbert A. Direske, Epidemiologist, Professor C. C. deSilva, Pediatrician, and Dr. J. Gulasekeram, Bacteriologist, all of Ceylon. While in East Pakistan, Dr. T. Guthe, World Health Organization, suggested an expansion of my ideas on the treponematoses and helped the production of the article forming the chapter on that subject.

After being rejected by more than thirty editors, the paper on evolution was finally accepted by Dr. Marti Ibanez for publication in the *International Record of Medicine* through the agency of Mr. Marcus Rosenblum, Editor of Public Health Reports. Mr. Rosenblum has edited several of my papers for me.

The ideas on eradication arose while Advisor in Health to the Government of East Pakistan for the International Cooperation Administration during the great epidemics of smallpox and cholera in East Pakistan in 1958. For the duration of the emergency, I was gazetted Director of the Institute of Public Health, Dacca, and appointed executive Deputy Chairman of the Epidemic Control Committee. International teams from the U.S.S.R., Afghanistan, International Cooperation Administration, U.S. Navy (NMRU2), and the Communicable Disease Center, United States Public Health Service, came to assist and I wish to acknowledge that much information was obtained from the members of these teams. I learned much about cholera and smallpox from the physicians of East Pakistan. Mr. James G. Cassanos and Mr. Richard Towle of International Cooperation Administration provided valuable help.

In 1960, the Johns Hopkins University School of Hygiene and Public Health and the National Institutes of Health provided me with a Fellowship through the support of Dr. Ernest L. Stebbins and Dr. Joseph E. Smadel. During the nine months in Baltimore, the papers on eradication and the species concept in microbiology were prepared. The criticisms of Dr. Philip E. Sartwell and his staff were of great value. A debt of gratitude is due to Dr. Eugene P. Campbell, Dr. Roy Fritz, and the staff of the Health Section, Agency for International Development in Washington, who not only provided data and criticism, but also arranged a special meeting with their consultants to discuss the paper on eradication. The support of the experts at this meeting, and in particular, Dr. Louis L. Williams, Pan American Health Bureau, was instrumental in having the paper accepted for publication in *Science*.

Professor G. S. Wilson, London, and Dr. Peter Mattingley, British Museum, are friends of the past twenty years who have given freely of their time and experience in supplying information and advice. Dr. Mattingley gave me my first instruction on mosquitoes at the Army School of Hygiene, Aldershot Command in 1942 and continued this during the two years we served together in West Africa. He supplied the information on fossil insects. Professor J. B. Cleland graciously supplied copies of his papers on diseases of Australian aborigines. Dr. Robert J. Huebner, National Institutes of Health, has been a constant source of information, criticism, and support for many years; and he and his colleagues at the National Institutes have been unstinting in their help. In 1958, Dr. Huebner organized a seminar at the National Institutes of Health to discuss my ideas.

In Cincinnati, I am deeply indebted to the Commissioner of Health, Dr. Kenneth I. E. Macleod, for his unfailing support and sympathy. The work on the eradication of syphilis, tuberculosis, and poliomyelitis in Cincinnati was done in the closest collaboration with him. Dr. Herman Nimitz and Mr. Kenneth Curfman have also assisted in Cincinnati. Dr. Fred L. Soper, for whose work on eradication I have the greatest respect, has frequently given me good advice.

Significant contribution of data and criticism were provided by the following: Dr. P. R. Edwards and Dr. Joan Taylor (*Salmonellae*),

Dr. Richard Thompson (Bacteriology), Dr. Albert B. Sabin (Virology), Dr. Philips Thygeson (Ophthalmology), Dr. Henry N. Russell (Astronomy), Dr. Ida Mann (Trachoma in Australia), Dr. Guido Crocetti and Dr. Owsei Temkin. Miss Juanita McBee helped with the preparation of the final draft and typed out the completed manuscript.

To all these fellow workers and many more not listed above, I am deeply indebted.

Nothing in this list of acknowledgments is to be taken to imply that any of the named scientists have in any way endorsed my ideas. In fact many were in full disagreement with the conclusions I drew from their data. With true scientific spirit, they helped in spite of their disagreements.

AIDAN COCKBURN

Cincinnati, Ohio
May, 1963

Contents

CHAPTER 1

The Role of Speculation
in Research

MUCH OF THE reasoning and thought in this work is of the type dismissed by most epidemiologists as "philosophic" or "mere speculation." In the field of infectious disease there is a profound distrust of speculation in most of its forms and, indeed, uncontrolled flights of fancy can lead to disastrous conclusions. However, possibly science is suffering from reaction to the speculative excesses of the Middle Ages when philosophers could gravely debate the number of angels that could dance on the point of a needle. Perhaps the reaction has gone too far.

My own experience of this distrust of speculation is such that I regard a defense of its use in research as essential, and the first chapter of this book will be devoted to this one point.

Three incidents described below tell of the potential fruitfulness of fancy in the fields of malaria, the treponematoses, and encephalitis, followed by one failure just to emphasize that more speculations fail than succeed.

In West Africa in 1942–44, malaria was the major public health problem so far as British Army troops were concerned. Within the past few years it has become clear that certain forms of primate malaria are readily transmittable to man by mosquitoes, but this was not known during World War II. The chimpanzees of West Africa have a *Plasmodium* that is indistinguishable morphologically from a human form, and the possibility was considered that such a parasite might be transmissible to man and of importance in a local way in the epidemiology of human malaria. The idea was encouraged by the late Brigadier G. M. Findlay, at that time Consultant in Medicine in West Africa, who stated that some forms of monkey malaria in India had already been transmitted to man. After the war, I encountered the theory that related hosts often have related or identical parasites. The way was now clear to expound the speculation that primate and human malarias had descended in quite recent time from a common ancestor, and that the primate infection might be of considerable importance in the maintenance of the human one. This opinion was expressed in a paper, but was promptly rejected by the journal to which it was submitted on the grounds that it was completely unfounded and without experimental support. In 1953 I finished a book in which similar concepts were developed for other infectious diseases; by 1959, this had been rejected in whole, part, or summary by more than thirty publishers or editors of journals. With only a few exceptions, the reviewers stated that the work was interesting, but too unsubstantial, too speculative, too imaginative, and without firm factual or experimental support. Finally, Dr. Robert J. Huebner invited a presentation of the basic concepts to a group at the National Institutes of Health in 1958, and for this purpose a summary draft was prepared that cut out some of the more unacceptable points, including the possibility that primate malaria might be of importance to the human disease. This presentation led to the discovery of an editor who was bold enough to accept the MS for publication, thus a summary of my ideas on evolution finally appeared (1). Two years later, a chance laboratory accident revealed that some primate malarias are in fact easily transmissible to man (2), and now great sums of money and scientific time are being devoted to the matter.

A second such point, also omitted from the published draft, had a more fortunate fate. In discussing the treponemes, the suggestion was made that they must have descended from a free-living form, since all parasites have been derived in this fashion. Furthermore, such a form might well be living today. The success of the general article on evolution encouraged me to work on a more specialized one on the treponematoses. With the assistance of Dr. T. Guthe, WHO Geneva, this was completed and included the concept of a free-living treponeme. This ran into the usual opposition of reviewers who did not like "unjustifiable speculation," but finally appeared in print (3). Within a few months of publication, a free-living form of treponeme had been reported (4), which had the Reiter antigen common to all the other parasitic treponemes (5). It has been given the name of *Treponema zuelzerae*.

Both the recognition of the transmissibility of primate malaria to man and the finding of the free-living treponeme were chance events that might have taken many years to occur. The discoveries could have been made much more quickly and surely had speculation from basic principles been used as a basis for experiments and surveys.

Because of the undeserved criticism of this way of working, such opportunities are frequently lost. Imagination is an essential ingredient in research, and speculation is the yeast that lightens the heavy dough of facts, making them palatable and easily digestible. It can act as a kind of catalyst or enzyme, speeding up the thought processes that lead to true discovery.

My favorite example of a rejected speculation is that of Lumsden's on the 1933 epidemic of encephalitis in St. Louis. In the summer of that year, this city was afflicted with a mysterious new infection, affecting thousands of people and causing many deaths and much disability. It created such alarm, nearing panic proportions in some sections, that many teams of scientists converged on the city. The disease was quickly described, the pathology elucidated, and the causal virus isolated. Only one thing remained to be discovered for control of the epidemic, the means of spread of the virus. One investigator, Dr. Lumsden, doing orthodox shoe-leather epidemiology, speculated that the virus was transmitted by mosquitoes and produced field data to support this idea. The others could not agree on the mechanism of transmission except on the one point that it was not by mosquitoes.

A comprehensive report which excluded mosquito transmission was signed by no less than eighty distinguished scientists, and this appeared as a monograph in Public Health Reports (6). Lumsden wrote a one-man minority report in favor of mosquito transmission, but this was not published and existed only in manuscript form. In 1948 at the Encephalitis Investigations Unit, U.S.P.H.S., the mosquito transmission of St. Louis encephalitis virus was accepted by all workers: the eighty-man majority report was regarded as little more than an interesting piece of history, while Lumsden's manuscript was passing from hand to hand, with fresh copies constantly being typed. Lumsden had the satisfaction of knowing, before he died in 1946, that his speculations were being accepted, and justice was finally done when his paper of 1933 was published in Public Health Reports in 1958 (7).

The example of a failure deals with appendicitis. Appendicitis first came to my notice in 1935 within a few months of leaving medical school; while practicing in Bedlington, Northumberland, England, six cases appeared in a street in one week where there had been none for many years, and a similar event occurred a few months later in another street. These looked like epidemics, and the possibility that appendicitis might be an infectious disease was stored away in my mind. In 1941, while Deputy Assistant Director of Hygiene, Aldershot Command, outbreaks of upper respiratory infections and pneumonias were reported from the girls' camps of the Auxiliary Territorial Service located in the Command. There were about 8,000 girls scattered in numerous camps, and in some places as many as 40 per cent had been ill. Some of the girls had had merely sore' throats, with the tonsils red and swollen, but a percentage of this group also complained of severe abdominal pain. About 120 such cases were reported, so a detailed study was made of one of the camp areas situated in Camberley, where there had been no appendicitis during the previous year. Twenty girls there had had abdominal pain of a more severe nature and had been under observation for possible appendicitis. Six had been admitted to the Louise Margaret Hospital, Aldershot, and laparotomies performed. Four had inflamed appendices, one had inflamed and swollen mesenteric glands, and one only free fluid in the abdomen with a normal appendix.

My report of an outbreak of an appendicitis-like infectious disease was not favorably received by Army medical circles; the various consultants expressed complete disbelief in my reasoning which was dismissed as being farfetched and unfounded speculation.

The discovery of the enteroviruses and adenoviruses has now permitted the whole picture of such diseases to be reopened, and the idea that some forms of appendicitis may be infectious diseases is now considered as a distinct possibility. It was with interest that I read recently the report of an outbreak in New York of a strange appendicitis-like disease almost identical with the one studied so many years ago in Aldershot (8).

In Cincinnati in 1961, the opportunity of testing this idea presented itself. With the assistance of surgeons and a pathologist, 20 appendices showing inflammation were collected and tested for enteroviruses and adenoviruses by Dr. Leon Rosen, National Institutes of Health, Bethesda, Maryland. No virus was isolated. It had seemed a good idea, but it just did not work out. Such a failure has to be taken philosophically: for every success, there are many of these.

There are various ways in which scientific discoveries can be made. The easiest, merely to observe a phenomenon and describe it, has its values, for enough observations may accumulate to make obvious some design or order underlying the mass of data.

Another way is to have one's mind educated and prepared in a particular field so that when some unusual opportunity arises, it will be grasped and recognized for what it is. In microbiology, there have been many examples, such as the unexpected finding by Huebner and Rowe of adenoviruses while growing adenoidal material in tissue culture (9); this could easily have passed unrecognized had not the workers been mentally prepared to appreciate the phenomenon when it occurred. Other findings are made by chance, as when the ship of a sailor is blown off course and he makes land at some unknown coast, as did the Norsemen, who found the New World while looking for Greenland.*

The Greeks relied chiefly on a combination of observations, assumptions, and deductions. This method, which is associated with the name of Aristotle, consists of taking some basic postulates and arguing step by step from them to attain some unassailable conclusion. This method has come in for severe criticism. According to Jeans, "Aristotle is generally credited with the invention of formal logic—the logic of rigorous proof—and some think this was an even greater disaster to science than his physics. He was right in insisting that no fact could be certain unless it had been deducted by strict logic from other facts which were certainly true, but he failed to see that this is just what we can never do in science. . . . As his premises were almost invariably wrong, his conclusions were so likewise" (10).

The method of induction, in which the argument is from the particular to the general, and reliance on experimentation, dates back to Bacon and Leonardo da Vinci.

The model way of making discoveries is to be ready to use all methods; to observe, to be well informed, to be mentally alert, and therefore ready to seize on opportunity that chance puts in one's way. Deduction, induction, or experimentation can then be used as the occasion requires. Yet these can be slow ways of making progress, and the catalyst of imagination serves to speed up the process. It is at this point that the term "speculation" tends to be used and that is where most scientists become uneasy and increasingly critical. The ideal approach to any problem is to begin with solid facts, from these draw certain irreproachable deductions, and in turn use these deductions to reach a firm and unassailable conclusion that can be confirmed by experiment or further observation.

* My own experience of a chance discovery is as follows:
While hunting elephant in West Africa in 1943, I was bitten on the leg by a tse-tse fly and developed a sore at the site. Trypanosomes were demonstrated in the lesion. At the urging of Dr. C. M. Wenyon, an account of the incident was published (Cockburn, T. A.: Case of Severe Reaction to Antrypol. Trans. Roy. Soc. Trop. Med. Hyg., 1947, 40, No. 4). This has proved to be the first description of what is now known as the Trypanosomal chancre in African sleepy sickness.

This is the method (except for the experimental confirmation) used successfully by Darwin to drive home his theory on evolution by natural selection (11). Many predecessors had attempted something similar, but had failed to buttress their arguments with the required foundation of fact and logic. Darwin began with two facts; first, he said that all organisms tend to increase in number in geometric fashion; and second, in spite of this, the numbers of a given species in a certain environment remain more or less constant. These are matters of everyday observances to any naturalist and are beyond dispute. From this, he deduced that therefore in nature a "struggle for existence" must occur in which either the majority of organisms die before reproducing themselves or else their full reproductive potential is not attained. Now came the third fact that all organisms vary appreciably. This together with the previous deduction permitted a further deduction: a form of natural selection must operate in which those individuals best adapted to their environment will survive and those less adapted will be eliminated—i.e. "the survival of the fittest." Now comes the fourth fact, that a great deal of variation is inherited, and this leads to the conclusion that the effects of differential survival will accumulate from generation to generation so that natural selection will thus act continually to improve the adjustment of organisms to their surroundings.

This is a classic example of the marriage of fact and logic, and when Darwin supported his conclusion with numerous examples from nature, the final acceptance of his theory was almost inevitable. The only flaw is in the term "survival of the fittest" which is a circular one, since the fittest are of course those that survive. Incidentally, Darwin did not include references to microbiology in his *On the Origin of Species,* but it is quite easy to apply his technique and demonstrate that his conclusions hold in that field as well as for the plants and animals. Yet Darwin's theory is based upon deduction and faces the same hazards as those of Aristotle in that it makes certain tacit assumptions which are not acceptable to many people. As a result, the theory is still only one of several, in spite of its seemingly irresistible logic. Simpson (12), in discussing the relations of great philosophic problems to evolution, states, "These questions are always approached on the basis of a prior postulate, seldom frankly stated, often nonscientific and sometimes even anti-scientific. In the Soviet Union, purely political postulates forced support of Michurinism, a form of Neo-Lamarckism, even though most Russian biologists knew all the time that accumulated evidence has made that theory extremely improbable. Orthodox Christian, and particularly Roman Catholic, postulates are often, but not necessarily, construed as demanding vitalistic and finalistic control of evolution." To people with such basic postulates, Darwin's arguments make no more appeal than Aristotle's on physics did to Sir James Jeans.

Any argument or reasoning process has to begin, either openly or tacitly, by making a number of assumptions. For example, Euclid prefaced his book on geometry with a number of axioms which were held to be obviously correct so that no proof of their correctness was needed. At the time they looked perfectly reasonable, but now it is doubtful if any of these would satisfy the astronomers in this era of relativity and curved space. Many so-called axioms, "facts," postulates, and assumptions that are self-evident in one time and place are not so self-evident in another, so that all conclusions derived from reasoning based on these have to be checked and cross-checked at frequent intervals.

In this attempt to outline the evolution of the infectious diseases, there are great difficulties in producing both facts and suitable methods of reasoning and argument: not only are there all the limitations of the science of paleontology, but also the handicap that at present there are almost no records of bacteria and viruses in the form of fossils. However, recent progress has shown algae and other primitive forms of life in strata laid down as long ago as two billion years, as described in Chapter 3. Such data are largely for the future, and at the present time the only lines of approach to the problems are those of comparative morphologies of the parasites and their hosts, and analogies between conditions and diseases of today and those of the past.

It has been pointed out that deductions from comparative morphology and modern analogy cannot be confirmed by experiment. If someone should contend (as has been done) that the ichthyosaurs, the whales, and the ratites or flightless birds are all descended from a common stock, then there is no sure way of proving or disproving the opinion. Similarly, if it is claimed, as in a later paper in this book, that the malaria parasite *Plasmodium* is descended from a free-living protozoon, then the matter cannot be proved or disproved experimentally. Even if it were demonstrated in the laboratory that it could be done, this would only show that it was possible and not that it actually happened, for as yet there is no fossil record either of *Amoeba* or *Plasmodium*. While it is possible to argue with Le Gros Clark that paleontology might almost be called an experimental science if "experiment" be defined as in the Oxford Dictionary as a "procedure adopted for testing a hypothesis" (13), yet in the field of paleoepidemiology even this cannot apply, since the lack of fossils does not permit us to test our hypothesis. (One unkind critic has defined prehistory as the "study of the unverifiable to prove the unwarrantable about what never happened anyway.")

The most reliable data come from our knowledge of infectious diseases today: by analogy, we can attempt to portray the diseases and infections of animals of past eras. There is much difference of opinion on the reliability of this method. One of its leading proponents was Wood Jones (14) who thought that it was at least as good as the evidence produced by the geologic record. He recalled that the workers who described the evolution of the horse, using fossils to illustrate the various steps, did it correctly, but by error used fossil horses that were not in the correct line of descent. The task could have been done just as well by using analogies with existing animals. Le Gros Clark supports this, saying, "It is particularly noteworthy how closely some of the fossil types conform to intermediate stages that had been postulated on the evidence of comparative anatomy. Discoveries of such fossil relics, indeed, provide a remarkable vindication of the well-established methods of comparative morphology. . . ." (13). On the other hand, Hooten (15) replies that this is not true. For example, early man walked upright but had a small brain, and since no such creature exists at the present time, no amount of reasoning by analogy could have inferred his existence. In the study of infections, such reasonings are largely academic, since all we have is the method of analogy, although some day it may be possible to demonstrate ancient infections with some certainty.

In my own research into fields where facts are few, speculation has played a large part and has been very productive in producing concepts that have later been confirmed by investigation and experiment. It must be emphasized that speculation is a matter of necessity and not choice, for where enough facts are at hand, logic can be employed. Out of my mistakes over the years I have developed a form of self-discipline and have drawn upon a series of mental rules. These have been useful in creating speculations that might lead to the discovery of new facts. They are as follows:

1. Wherever possible, search for the highest quality evidence. The finest evidence is always the best.
2. Begin by arguing from the basic principle to the particular, as did Aristotle, but if cross-checking by experiment or observa-

tion suggests some irregularity, then restudy the general principle
as well as the particular example.

3. If fact and theory to not agree, check the "fact" as well as
theory.

4. Avoid overspecialization and be well informed of work
in fields outside that under study.

5. Having set up a speculation, and assembled and arranged
arguments in support of it, reverse the process to assume that it
is not true, and see if even better arguments can be produced in
favor of the converse.

6. Avoid emotional attachment to one's ideas.

7. Before settling down to the technicalities of some specific
point, first try to visualize the total pattern in which the point
is located, and as research progresses, remain oriented by referring back to this pattern. Unless this is done, it is very easy to be
misled by some minor flaw in technique and end up with an
absurd result.

The finest evidence is the best.   This is a requirement of British
law, so that a court will not accept a photograph of a document if the
original itself can be produced. In the field of epidemiology, an
antibody has much the same relation to an antigen as the photo has
to the original document; it is good evidence of infection but not the
best.

In 1950, when engaged in field research into the ecology of Western Equine encephalomyelitis virus (WEE) in Colorado (16), a decision had to be made whether to rely upon antibody tests or virus
isolations for indications of infection. At that time the picture of
WEE infection in nature was very confused, with bird mites being
regarded as the main reservoirs of the virus, transmission to birds
occurring in the summer months, resulting in infection of mosquitoes
and possibly other biting arthropods, with subsequent spread by
these to many forms of vertebrates. This concept was to some extent
based on antibody tests on vertebrate sera, for these were relatively
cheap, costing only about $10.00 each. On the other hand, virus iso-
lations could run into big money. Only one isolation from a bird in
nature had ever been made, from a prairie chicken during the big
epidemic in North Dakota in 1941 (17).

On the general principle of always going for the best evidence, it
was decided to adopt virus isolation techniques for the demonstration of infection in birds. This was criticized on the grounds that
while it was theoretically desirable, it was not practical. Viraemia in

a bird lasts only about three to five days and, since birds like pigeons can live for ten years or more, the chances of bleeding one in the field while the virus was in its blood would be about one in ten thousand, so small that it makes the attempt not worth the effort and cost. However, the idea was tried out and was so successful that in 1951 no fewer than 11 isolations of WEE virus were made from 696 wild birds. Now, this technique is generally accepted and such isolations are routine. What was achieved by the isolation of virus was the certain knowledge of its presence at a certain time in a certain bird at a precise location. Compare this with the observation that a particular bird had antibodies against this virus. There would be no certainty that the antibodies had been caused by any particular virus, since other viruses with common antigens might have caused them, and indeed they might have been the result of infection with some virus not yet discovered. It would not be known when the infection had occurred, for some birds live for many years, nor could the location of infection be discovered, for a migrant bird could have acquired the infection thousands of miles away. If it were a very young bird, it might not have been infected at all, but have absorbed the antibodies from the yolk of the egg in which it developed and so have inherited them from the mother bird.

In the long run, it pays to go after the very best evidence available.

Basic principle to specific example. If a basic principle is applied to a situation, very often it can lead to a valuable finding. If it does not seem to fit the situation, it is either wrongly applied or the principle is not so basic and correct as one had thought, in which case the matter is worth further investigation. A principle that I have used a good deal in speculation is Darwin's concept of natural selection. From this, it follows that an organism is shaped by its environment within the limits of heredity and mutation, and therefore an organism with some accentuated feature may have a factor in the environment to account for it. The danger in this reasoning is that the feature may be secondary to another which may not be so obvious.

The point can be illustrated with the example of the giraffe and its long neck, which has intrigued zoologists since the days of Lamarck. Lamarck theorized that the neck grew long as a result of succeeding generations of giraffes constantly straining to reach leaves at the top of the trees. Darwinists did not like this idea of the inheritance of acquired characteristics, and said that, on the contrary, the neck was the result of natural selection, for in difficult times only those with the longest necks would survive and the others would die off. Both ignored the fact that females are often shorter than the males by one or two feet, while juveniles are shorter still. Under either theory, in a period of drought and starvation, there would be only adult males surviving; and giraffes would become extinct. The long neck is in fact secondary to long legs. Long legs have substantial survival value in most orders of mammals or birds both for defense and to escape, but all that acquire them have the same trouble of feeding or drinking from the ground. The elephant has overcome this problem with its trunk, the tapir with its proboscis, the ostrich with its long neck, and the heron and stork with a combination of long neck and beak. The giraffe's neck is no longer than is absolutely necessary to permit the animal to drink, as must be obvious to anyone who has seen the difficulty it has in spreading its front legs far enough apart to allow its tongue to reach the water. A neck has evolved that is long enough to keep pace with the lengthening legs; the males protect the females and young.

I recently had occasion to apply this form of thinking to the cholera vibrio. The most outstanding feature in the biology of this vibrio is its capacity to withstand a high level pH of the order of 10.0 or higher, and it can grow in a pH of 9.5. Most intestinal bacilli cannot exist for more than a few hours in such an environment, so it is natural to wonder what environmental factor could be responsible for selecting such a characteristic. Since there is no location within the body where such a pH is found, it must be somewhere outside the body. At that time, I was working in East Pakistan, where cholera is endemic. It is a very flat land, barely above sea level, flooded during the monsoon season, and short of drinking water during the dry season. Each village is surrounded by artificial ponds or tanks that are the sole supply of water for about eight months of the year, and where, in the course of the day, the entire population of the village comes to wash, bathe, clean clothes, wash down the cattle, fish, and collect water for drinking and cooking. Sometimes a latrine will be perched at one end. These tanks form an ideal arrangement for the exchange of intestinal organisms among the villagers, and must be the main agent of spread of the cholera vibrio. The environmental factor selecting the pH resistant characteristic in the vibrio would be most likely to be in the water of the tank. A quick test with a portable pH meter soon showed that the water in the tanks did at times have a pH as high as 10.0, but that it was extremely variable, being very low when the sky was cloudy and high during bright sunshine. Examination of the water in a series of tanks at different times of the day over a period of a year showed that such a cycle of pH changes did exist, and the studies provided an explanation not only for the epidemiology of cholera but also for the pH characteristic of the vibrio. This work is given in more detail in Chapter 8.

If fact and theory do not agree, check both fact and theory.   One of the commonest fallacies among epidemiologists is that the findings of the laboratory are facts, while conclusions drawn from observations in the field are only theories. Not only do all laboratory techniques have margins of error—and in some instances error can be substantial—but also the personal factor for variation is great, so that I have learned by experience to regard all laboratory reports as suspect until tested out in practice. Also, it is a mistake to reject one's theory on the basis of a so-called fact supported by work of some other scientist. Such a "fact" may be work showing that a certain organism is the causal agent of the disease under question, or that an insect is the transmitting agent of a particular pathogen. In several instances where the accepted data or the laboratory results did not fit with speculations, further study has proved the existence of some error in the former. Such an example occurred while I was working in West Africa on mosquitoes. Specimens were sent to a laboratory for testing by the precipitin test for the source of origin of the blood in the mosquitoes' stomachs, and a substantial proportion of the reports came back labeled "horse blood." This did not fit my ideas at all, but the laboratory scientists protested indignantly when their results and techniques were questioned. It was not until it was demonstrated that this was tsetse fly country and there was not a horse within a hundred miles of the location that the laboratory rechecked the technique used and found that an error in the cleaning of the pipettes had been giving false positives. Had there been horses in this region, it would have been difficult to convince the laboratory workers that they were in error.

In 1951, it was reported that the virus of Epidemic Keratoconjunctivitis (EKC), known as the Sanders EKC virus, was identical to that of St. Louis Encephalitis virus (18). This raised the possibilities either that the accepted concepts of the epidemiologies of these two infections were incorrect, or that the one virus caused the two diseases, or that something was wrong with the viruses. Naturally, the first to be checked were the theories, but what was known about the arthropod-borne viral encephalitides seemed reasonable apart from the role of mites. Since there was no first hand experience of EKC, a small epidemic that came conveniently to hand was investigated, and the findings confirmed what was already reported in the literature (19), i.e., the infection was spread largely by infected instruments in ophthalmologists' offices. It seemed most unlikely that two infections, the epidemiologies of which were so different, could be caused by a common agent, so attention was turned to the viruses. The experience of our unit with St. Louis encephalitis virus was consistent with the idea that this was, in fact, the causal agent of the disease, so attention was next paid to what at that time was also generally accepted as a fact—that the Sanders EKC virus was the causal agent of that disease.*

The investigation took two forms, study of the material from the epidemic and a review of the history of the virus. Convalescent sera from the cases of EKC in the epidemic investigated proved to have no antibodies against either St. Louis or the Sanders EKC viruses. Presumably, therefore, this epidemic had not been caused by either virus. EKC virus had a peculiar history in that during the war all strains were lost except one; this one had been stored in the same deep freeze as St. Louis virus, and there had been opportunity for this one surviving strain to become contaminated with St. Louis virus during storage. It was therefore concluded that the Sanders EKC virus in existence was the contaminating strain of St. Louis virus and not related to the disease (20, 21). This conclusion has been abundantly confirmed by later demonstration that the disease EKC is caused by adenoviruses which are quite different from the so-called Sanders EKC virus.†

* The Sanders EKC virus was described in some detail as being the etiologic agent of the disease in the official *Army History of Preventive Medicine in World War II*, published in 1960. The fact that this work is no longer generally accepted is not mentioned in the text (*Preventive Medicine in World War II*, Vol. 5, Communicable Diseases, Medical Department, Office of the Surgeon General, Department of the Army, Washington).

† The studies in 1951 on the possible relationship between EKC and encephalitis led to the discovery of a new disease entity characterized by conjunctivitis, corneal opacities, muscle pain, pyrexia, and pharyngitis. This was called "Greeley Disease" (Cockburn, T. A.: An epidemic of conjunctivitis in Colorado: associated with pharyngitis, muscle pain and pyrexia. Am. J. Ophthal., 1953, **36**: 1534–39). Two years later, Huebner and his colleagues discovered the adenoviruses. Sera from the Greeley incident had been kept stored in the deep freeze, and when these were tested in 1954 against adenoviruses, rising titers of antibodies were demonstrated against Type 3 (Cockburn, T. A., Rowe, W. P., and Huebner, R. J.: Relationship of the 1951 Greeley Colorado outbreak of conjunctivitis and pharyngitis to Type 3 APC virus infection. Amer. J. Hyg., 1956, **63**: 250–53). The disease entity is now called pharyngo-conjunctival fever.

Avoid overspecialization. During the studies in encephalitis referred to above, and before the technique of virus isolation from birds had been developed, serologic tests were used to determine if virus was active in the test locality in any one season of the year. Baby birds were examined, on the grounds that since they were only a few weeks old, any antibodies in their blood must represent very recent infections and therefore current activity of the virus in the test area. The results of the first season's work quickly showed that many of the nestlings did in fact have antibodies against WEE virus, and considerable time was spent studying the nest ecology of these nestlings to see how the virus was being transmitted. Finally, some pigeon squabs only a few days old were found to have sera that had high titer antibodies, and only then did it occur to both the laboratory and field staff at the same time that the antibodies were coming through the egg from the mother and that the squabs had at no time been exposed to WEE virus (22). This finding not only invalidated our work on baby birds in that year but also cast doubt on the value of similar studies in other parts of the world. It also led to substantial changes in our laboratory techniques, for we were using day-old chicks for attempted isolations of virus. Since these chicks were hatched from fertile eggs bought locally, and the study area was deliberately chosen because WEE virus was active there, many of our day-old chicks would be immune to the virus as a result of this transovarian passage of antibodies.

This discovery of transovarian antibody passage not only pointed up the dangers in interpretation of serologic findings as mentioned above, but also showed that we were not familiar with the literature in related disciplines. The passage of antibodies through the egg had been known for more than half a century and had been demonstrated in a wide variety of infections. Had we been acquainted with this other work, through broader reading of the literature, our reasoning on the value of young birds as sentinels for the detection of virus activity, as well as for the isolation of virus in the laboratory, would have been very different.

A somewhat different situation arose during the cholera work in East Pakistan. By the middle of 1958, tests had shown that the tank waters around Dacca did in fact have marked shifts in the pH in the course of the day and that this would account for the epidemiology of cholera. In the normal way of research, one would then have gone to the nearest university, sought out a limnologist, and asked for advice. Such a person would have explained that it is well known that algae can change the pH in this fashion according to the light available. Unfortunately, in Dacca there was no person available for consultation, and further the library facilities were very inadequate, so that this information was not forthcoming. Luckily, at this moment, an article on the respiration of sea plants appeared in *Science* (23) and this stimulated speculation that perhaps the respiration of the algae in the tanks would be enough to alter the pH to the extent observed. Observation showed that the pH changes did correlate with the sunlight. My article was accepted for publication before I returned to the U.S.A.; it was with intense relief that it was found that the pH changes due to algae were common knowledge among limnologists, but the relief was mixed with annoyance that scientific isolation had forced the working out of facts already published in the literature.

Consider both the speculation and its converse. The process of reversing a speculation to see if the converse is the more likely can be illustrated by the example of the arthropod-borne infections. Until 1954, the speculation had been accepted uncritically in most of the scientific world that these originated in the arthropod and that the development of the vertebrate cycle came later.

A strong supporter of arthropod origin has been Hoare who, at a meeting just after World War II, stated that "at present most protozoologists accept Leger's theory of the evolution of the haemo-flagellates, according to which they have descended from the mono-genetic insect flagellates." In the discussion that followed, this view did not go unchallenged, for Dias stated that "the generally accepted Leger's theory on the origin of the Trypanosomidae finds it difficult to explain important biological facts that are easily explained by Minchin's theory. It seems possible that some digenetic flagellates now existing have originated from primitive parasites of vertebrates" (24). However, Dias seemed to be in a very small minority, for without exception, everyone with whom I have discussed the matter has agreed with Hoare. A leading exponent of arthropod origin has been Huff, who in 1938 had produced arguments in favor that had stood unrefuted ever since (25). In 1954, when I read Huff's paper, some of the arguments did not seem to ring true. Accordingly, acting on this method of reversing the hypothesis and so trying to prove the converse, an attempt was made to demonstrate how a parasite like *Plasmodium* could have evolved first in a vertebrate and spread to the mosquito at a later date.

Huff had speculated that the precursors of parasites like *Plasmo-dium* and *Rickettsia* had originally been parasites of arthropod intestines, so attention was paid to the vertebrate intestines to see if parasites similar to *Plasmodium* could be found there also. This was quickly found to be the case, and indeed one of these, *Eimeria*, had first provided the clue to the life cycle of *Plasmodium* because of the resemblances between them.

Intestinal organisms must gain frequent entry to the blood via the portal system, and so could easily be picked up by blood-sucking arthropods. This can be done directly, as happens in *Schellackia*, a parasite of snakes in which the cycle is a simple one of an intestinal infection of the snake, followed by a blood infection, ingestion by a mite, and swallowing of the mite by the snake. Most protozoa, however, seem to have colonized the liver first, this being the organ most easily reached from the intestine; and it can easily be speculated that spread to other parts of the body and to blood-sucking vertebrates followed from this. The process has been described in more detail later in this book under Theory 8 in the chapter on evolution.

As a result of reversing the speculation, in the case of *Plasmodium*, stronger case was made for vertebrate origin than for the original one.

Avoid emotional attachment to one's ideas. It is a fatal mistake to become so tied to a particular product of one's brain that the ability to see it in a detached fashion is lost. One then becomes emotionally the intellectual "mother" of this brain child, holding it to be the best of all children, perhaps in spite of some deformity obvious to all other "mothers." This has happened to me in the past, and caused so much pain that now I make a conscious effort to avoid this form of attachment. I know now that of any ten ideas that occur to me, perhaps as many as nine will be proved wrong. This no longer upsets me: I patiently follow up as many as possible and am not surprised when one after another trail reaches a dead end. The process has its rewards, for in looking for one thing, the mere act of research may reveal something else unsuspected and even more worth-while, just as in the case of Saul who went searching for his father's ass and found a kingdom. When the tenth idea proves correct, the total effort is amply repaid. With this kind of philosophy, it is possible to regard all one's ideas, theories, and speculations with a considerable degree of remoteness, to see deformities before being told of them, and to make the necessary corrections or discards.

However, after thinking hard on a problem or a paper for some considerable time, one's critical senses become fatigued. After reading the same lines and data over and over again, the words, figures, and charts cease to have any fresh meaning and tend to become hypnotic. This is the dangerous stage, and there are two methods of dealing with it. The first is to put away the manuscript for some months and work on something different; it is amazing how easy it is to spot obvious mistakes after returning with a fresh and clear mind to a paper laid aside for some time. The other method is the time-honored one of requesting, begging, persuading, and badgering experts in the field to criticize the work and listening carefully to what they have to say. This process is not one that makes new friends or keeps old ones, but it certainly improves one's work and avoids gross deformities from becoming obvious only after the Rubicon of publication has been crossed.

In spite of these safeguards, the tendency to have protective feelings for one's ideas does grow. Knowledge of my own failings in this respect has led me to have a warm regard for a certain old professor in Italy. He had taught Aristotle's ideas on science and astronomy all his life, and now a young upstart called Galileo, in his own university, was claiming to have invented a device called the telescope that proved Aristotle wrong. Galileo was saying that if you looked through this telescope, you could see that Jupiter had two moons. He was even asking everyone to come and look for themselves to see the moons with their own eyes. It was a trick of course. It must be. There are no moons there, or Aristotle would have said so. Still, better not look through that telescope or you might see these moons. And if you see them, what are you going to do? Can you confess, even to yourself, you have been teaching the untruth all your life?

The old professor shook his head and went back to his classroom and Aristotle, leaving Galileo looking through his telescope. He has my sympathy.

Speculation is a dangerous business in which there is no room for amateurs, beginners, and small boys. Anyone wishing to indulge in it should first ask himself if he has served a long enough apprenticeship in his trade and is fully master of his tools. It has much in common with bullfighting; the problem is the bull, and the tools are the cloak of imagination which maneuvers the bull to best advantage and the sword which is a delicate instrument of fact and experiment that must be plunged with skill, precision, and elegance into one tiny, hidden, yet vital spot.

Recently in Madrid, a novice bullfighter, about eighteen years old, played his bull magnificently for ten minutes, winding the beast slowly, gracefully, dangerously, around himself while the "oles" shook the plaza. But four times he tired to kill it and each time he failed. When finally the bull died, the boy laid his head on the *barrera* and cried and cried.

"Orteguita, crying yesterday against the barrera, dreams of being another Ordonez but Ordonez would not have wept over a failure. Ordonez is a pro and quite cynical. So are all other pros. If they do not feel well, if they do not like the look of the bull, they dispatch it at once, any way they can. The crowd throws cushions, and the matador leaves the ring stonyfaced, or sometimes, guarded by the police. He knows that tomorrow is another day; tomorrow he may or may not fight well. He does not weep. The pros don't weep in the bullfighting business" (26).

G. Udney Yule, that celebrated and hard-headed mathematician on whose handbook, introducing the useful and elusive subject of statistics, generations of budding students all over the world have cut their teeth, had definite views on speculation. One of his sayings on the subject was thought important enough to be included in his obituary in the list of Fellows of the Royal Society, and is so much in line with this chapter that it will be used to conclude it (27).

"If you get on the wrong track with mathematics for your guide, the only result is that you get to the Valley of Mare's Nests much quicker. Logic and Mathematics are only of service when once you have found the right track; and to find the right track you must exercise faculties quite other than the logical—Observation, and Fancy, and Imagination: accurate observation, riotous fancy, and detailed and precise imagination."

REFERENCES

1. COCKBURN, T. A.: The evolution of infectious diseases. Int. Rec. Med., 1959, **172**: 493–508.
2. EYLES, D. E., COATNEY, R. G., AND GETZ, M. E.: Simian malaria transmitted to man. Science, 1960, **131**: 1812.

3. COCKBURN, T. A.: The origins of the treponematoses. Bull. W.H.O., 1961, 24: 221–28.
4. VELDKAMP, H.: Isolation and characteristics of *Treponema zuelzerae* nov. species, an anaerobic free-living spirochaete. Antonie Leeuwenhoek, 1960, 26: 103–25.
5. DE BRUIJN, J. H.: Serologic relationships between *Treponema zuelzerae* and the Reiter strain of *T. pallidum*. Antonie Leeuwenhoek, 1961, 27: 98–102.
6. Report on the St. Louis outbreak of encephalitis. Public Health Bull., 1935, 214.
7. LUMSDEN, L. L.: St. Louis encephalitis in 1933. Public Health Rep., 1958, 73: 339–54.
8. McMAHON, D. P.: An unusual outbreak of disease in New York State. Morbidity & Mortality Weekly Reports. C.D.C., U.S.P.H.S., 1961, 10: No. 36, p. 2.
9. ROWE, W. P., et al.: Isolation of a cytopathogenic agent from human adenoids. Proc. Soc. Exp. Biol. & Med., 1953, 84: 570–73.
10. JEANS, SIR J.: *The Growth of Physical Science*. Cambridge Univ. Press, Cambridge, 1947.
11. DARWIN, C.: *On the Origin of Species*. John Murray, London, 1859.
12. SIMPSON, G. G.: Historical biology bearing on human origins, in Cold Spring Harbor Symp. XV, 1947.
13. LE GROS CLARK: *A History of the Primates*. Brit. Mus., London, 1949.
14. WOOD JONES, F.: *Man's Place Among the Mammals*. Edward Arnold, London, 1929.
15. HOOTEN, E. A.: *Up from the Ape*. Macmillan Co., New York, 1946.
16. COCKBURN, T. A., SOOTER, C. A., AND LANGMUIR, A. D.: The ecology of western equine and St. Louis encephalitis viruses. Amer. J. Hyg., 1957, 65: 130–46.
17. COX, H. R.: Isolation of western equine encephalo-myelitis virus from a naturally infected prairie chicken. Public Health Rep., 1941, 56: 1905–6.
18. RUCHMAN I.: Relationship between epidemic keratoconjunctivitis and St. Louis encephalitis viruses, Proc. Soc. Exp. Biol. Med., 1951, 77: 120–25.
19. COCKBURN, T. A., ROBINSON, T., NITOWSKY, H., AND CHEEVER, F. S.: Epidemic keratoconjunctivitis; a study of a small epidemic. Amer. J. Ophthal., 1953, 36: 1367–72.
20. COCKBURN, T. A.: Shipyard eye. Brit. Med. J., 1959, 2: 429–30.
21. COCKBURN, T. A.: The present status of epidemic keratoconjunctivitis. Amer. J. Ophthal., 1954, 38: 476–85.
22. SOOTER, C. A., SHAEFFER, M., GORRIE, R. AND COCKBURN, T. A.: Transovarian of antibodies following naturally acquired encephalitis infection in birds. J. Infect. Dis., 1954, 95: 165–67.
23. RYTHER, J. H.: The productivity of the sea. Science, 1959, 130: 602–8.
24. HOARE, C. A.: The relationships of the haemo flagellates. Proc. 4. Inter. Congr. on Trop. Med. & Malaria, Washington, 1948.
25. HUFF, C. G.: Studies on the evolution of some disease-forming organisms. Quart. Rev. Biol., 1938, 13: 196–206.
26. DALEY, R.: The pros don't cry in the bullfighting business. *New York Times*, Sept. 26, 1961.
27. YULE, G. UDNEY: quoted in Obituary Notices of Fellows of the Royal Society, 1952, 8: 313.

CHAPTER 2

Evolutionary Background

FOR A FULL appreciation of the following chapters on evolution and eradication of infectious disease, a knowledge of the basic principles of evolution is necessary. The assumption is made that anyone interested enough to attempt to read this book has had biology instruction at least to the high school level and therefore is acquainted with these fundamentals; should any reader feel any deficiency in this field, there are plenty of textbooks available to him, ranging from the twenty-year-old classic by Sir Julian Huxley *Evolution: a Modern Synthesis* (1), still unsurpassed in its field, to Romer's *The Vertebrate Story* (2). The purpose of this chapter is to fill in the gaps not covered by such textbooks: it deals chiefly with the origin of life, and the evolutions of hosts, pathogens, vectors, and environments. All such matters are highly relevant to an understanding of the ways by which the various infections arose and obtained their present natures and distributions.

The starting point is a brief discussion on Darwin's theory on the origin of species (3) as applied to microbiology. Bacteria were not known with familiarity in Darwin's day, and the viruses were not discovered until after his death, so were never mentioned in his book. Yet it is easy to show that the facts and deductions on which he based his theory of natural selection apply to microbiology as well as to larger creatures. These have already been mentioned in the previous chapter. Facts one and two state that all creatures tend to increase in number in geometrical fashion, but that in any stable situation, the number of the creatures present is constant within narrow limits. Figure 1 illustrates this, being a curve of the number of viable organisms in a culture of bacteria.

At the beginning there is no increase in numbers (lag phase), but the bacteria are very active and grow in size. The length of the lag phase depends on factors such as the youth of the culture from which the organisms were taken, the size of the inoculum, the composition of the medium, and the temperature. This lag phase is due to the cells' need to adapt themselves to the new medium and to

20

reactivate any enzymes that may have declined in the previous culture (4).

The next phase is one of full reproductivity (logarithmic growth), indicated by the straight rising line in the growth curve. This is the period of geometric growth. It terminates and reproduction practically ceases until the number of cells dying out equals that of the ones reproducing, and the population size remains stationary. Finally the viable population slowly tails off. The cessation of re-

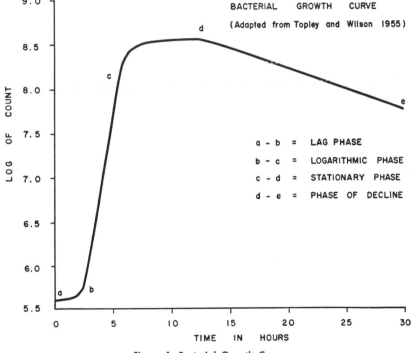

Figure 1. Bacterial Growth Curve.

production is sometimes considered due to the exhaustion of food and oxygen and the accumulation of poisonous waste particles, but it is found that if the culture is sterilized by heating, a fresh inoculum will grow almost as well as the first. Apparently there is a limiting concentration of organisms specific to each culture that cannot be exceeded.

That variation occurs in any culture of microorganisms is too well known to require any stress here. It is possible to start with a

WHITWORTH COLLEGE LIBRARY
SPOKANE, WASH.

single isolated microorganism and to rear a thousand million descendants in a short time. In that clone of organisms will be a host of mutants, covering a great range of variation. The frequency of each variant will depend on its nature, with perhaps about one per half million or so cell divisions being about the average, with extremes of about two or three powers in either direction. From these two facts, it follows that Darwin's deduction of a struggle for survival and the survival of the fittest will apply to such cultures as well as to large creatures. This means that every time a microorganism is introduced to a new and different culture medium, tissue culture tube, or host animal, the form of organism that will be selected, survive, and multiply in that new environment will be those best adapted to live there, and may be different from those predominating in the previous environment. Since much variation is inherited, the newly selected organism will become increasingly adapted to the new conditions.

All living creatures are divided into species and classified by this means. "Species" is difficult to define, and the accepted concept keeps changing; a few decades ago it meant a single type-specimen with which all other specimens were compared, but now it is defined usually as a population with a wide range of characters. For larger animals and plants, the standard definition of a species with this population concept emphasizes the importance of sexual interchange of genetic material. A widely quoted definition is that of Mayr: "Species are groups of actually or potentially interbreeding natural populations which are reproductively isolated from other such groups" (5). Since individual bacteria and viruses were thought until quite recently not to interbreed at all, but to multiply by various forms of fission, these definitions were simply not applicable to the microbiological world at large. In the last two decades, a vast change has taken place, and it has been demonstrated not only that actual mating of bacteria and protozoa takes place, but that genetic material is also transferred by viruses from one bacterium to another. In other words, the microorganisms are not unique, but like larger creatures can also share their genetic material within their specific populations. The result of this is to bring the microbiological world within the limits of the species definition of Mayr. A bacterial species, like that of larger creatures, is a population which is isolated from other species, in which genes are exchanged, and where individuals may show great variations. This is discussed in detail in a later chapter.

The modern classification of all the larger living things is phylogenetic in character; when a name is given to an organism, an attempt is made to locate that organism in its proper place in the evolutionary tree. The generic name implies that all species in the genus are descended from one common ancestor, just as all genera in a family are similarly descended from one ancestor and so on all through the various groupings of living organisms. To apply these concepts to an organism like the treponemes, all species of the genus *Treponema* must be regarded as having been descended from one ancestral species, and all species in the genus are potentially interbreeding groups that are reproductively isolated from one another.

If one species invaded a number of different environments, the selections made by the differing environments from the great mass of individuals within the population would vary from one place to another, but interbreeding between the groups and the sharing of genetic material would cancel out differences to a large extent. If the interbreeding were prevented by any form of isolation, then locally the differences would accumulate. As a result, the original population would "radiate" into new strains, and eventually new species would evolve. The isolation that would cause this interruption of interbreeding could be of various kinds, of which the most important would be geographical isolation, where the populations of the organisms are physically removed from one another, and ecological isolation, where they live in the same geographical location but where by reason of habit they do not come into contact with one another. In this fashion, geographical and ecological isolations lead to an "adaptive radiation" from a single common stock. The possibility that the treponemes have "radiated" in this fashion in response to geographical and ecological isolations is described in a later chapter.

All evolutionary change is based on inherited variation. The variations come by mutations, the distribution through the population being through the various forms of genetic spread mentioned earlier. When it is realized that in one single yaws lesion there are very many millions of organisms, each with many genes, it is obvious that in that lesion in the course of a single day very many mutations must appear, and that throughout the world the total daily count of mutations in treponemes must be colossal. The vast majority of these will die out, some because they themselves are lethal to their hosts, and others because they cannot stand the competition in the struggle for existence. So long as the environment stays unchanging, the pre-

dominant organisms will be those chosen by previous selective processes, and these will be better fitted to survive than the majority of
newly arriving mutants; as a result the chance of any new mutant
becoming established and replacing the existing ones is extremely
remote. Some mutants will survive if they cause no handicap. When,
however, the environment changes, the position is different. Existing
predominant genes may be at a disadvantage in the new conditions
and may be liable to be replaced by mutants already existing in the
gene pool or being created *de novo*. Such an environmental change
could be the invasion of an unusual host animal or type of tissue,
a new means of spread, the migration of the host to a fresh climate,
or the adoption of new customs. When this happens, provided the
organism is isolated from the main mass of genes, a new strain of
parasite evolves.

All attempts to trace back the origins of bacteria and viruses take
us back in the end to the question of the origin of life. This is a
highly technical and debated matter requiring training in basic
sciences that I do not possess, yet without some working hypothesis
on this point, a beginning cannot be made on this subject of the
evolution of infectious disease. My reading and contact with scientists
working in this area has produced such a working hypothesis that
this is now presented here without any attempt being made to justify
it. Probably many will disagree with individual features, yet as far
as I can determine, the main lines are in accordance with modern
thinking.

The Universe is about five billion years old. As cooling took
place, seas were formed, consisting of water that was only slightly
saline. The salinity increased to its present degree as the rivers washed
salt down from the lands. The original atmosphere of the world
consisted chiefly of ammonia, methane, carbon dioxide and similar
chemicals, and water vapor. The electrical storms common at that
time converted some of these into amino acids and other substances
required for the original synthesis of life. That this could happen
was demonstrated in the classic experiment of Miller working in
Urey's laboratory (6) in 1953, when amino acids were produced
through the agency of electric discharges from a mixture of gases
thought to be present under primitive earth conditions. Once it was
thought that the presence of oxygen was a necessity for the appearance
of life, but now it is generally accepted that oxygen was created in
its present abundance by life, rather than the other way round. If

all life disappeared from earth, the existing oxygen would soon disappear, being combined by the various partially oxidized rocks such as volcanic lava. A little would be formed in the upper atmosphere by the disintegration of water vapor into its atomic constituents under the influence of ultra violet light; the lighter hydrogen part of this would tend to escape from the earth's gravitational field, leaving behind the oxygen part. This, however, would be only a small fraction compared with that created by the photosynthesis of plants.

The idea of life originating in a "reducing atmosphere" was first proposed by Loebsack in 1912 (7), but it was the pioneering work of Oparin in 1937 (8) that first put such an anaerobic concept on an acceptable basis. Now the majority opinion seems to be that a form of biologic "soup" developed in the oceans of the earth, this containing a mixture of amino acids and other precursors of proteins and of DNA.

There is no unanimity on the manner in which these precursors combined to form more complex combinations. Oparin suggests a process called coazervation, but a number of other mechanisms have been proposed. For the purpose of this book, it is immaterial as to which one was correct, so long as it is accepted that at one time life evolved in the waters of the earth in the form of tiny discrete concentrates of substances not unlike naked genes or very simple viruses in size and composition.

It was supposed that during this period of "pre-life," some particles would break up and their components would be incorporated in others, thereby causing a constant state of interchange of substances. Those particles, which by chance had acquired the more efficient catalysts, would grow in size and complexity at the expense of those without them: this process of interchange of materials and catalysts would be of prime importance in the origin of "life." This would be of value later in the evolution of higher forms, with the catalysts now elevated to the status of enzymes. The simplest forms of exchange—that of breakdown and incorporation into other particles —would have survived to the present day in the process of transformation. On a larger scale, the union of two complete particles drawn together by the possession of unlike electric charges would be even more efficient; at this level, the particles would be somewhat of the dimensions and organization of "free-living" viruses and this would be the origin of transduction. Later, as the ocean's supplies of building materials became exhausted, being concentrated in the particles, some of the larger particles would evolve their own micro-climates in the nature of cytoplasm-containing envelopes that would approximate to some extent the conditions in the oceans of the primitive earth. This, however, would lead to difficulties in the transfer of substances between one organism and another. The simpler methods of transformation and transduction would still be of value and would continue in spite of the evolution of sexual means of exchange.

One of the big problems facing any study on the evolution of infectious disease is that of the origin of virus. The prevailing theory, first expounded by Laidlaw (9), is that they are largely degenerated intracellular parasitic bacteria, and indeed a very good case can be made for such an origin for many of the larger ones and especially the rickettsial and psittacosis groups. Yet it is becoming increasingly obvious that many viruses are not just simple parasites, but can also carry genetic material from one host cell to another. They may easily play an important role in the normal life of the cell, and therefore, must be considered as far more than parasites. Since there must at one time have been free-living "organisms" or at least preliving chemical complexes in the biologic soup that were of the same dimensions and basic chemical composition as present day viruses, I would like to think that some of these survived and are present today as our smaller viruses. Of course, they are free living only for a brief period in their life cycles, since the conditions in the environments have changed. The rest of their lives possibly is spent in a mutualistic association with those of their fellows that have evolved cytoplasmic coats, this association being usually of benefit to both.

MAN, THE HOST

Man belongs to the radiation of the primates. The living primates can be divided first into three main groups: the lemurs or prosimians; *Tarsius,* a curious rat-like creature from Indonesia with large eyes and some human features, intermediate between the lemurs and the higher primates; and the anthropoids which include monkeys and the higher apes. These are all believed to have descended from one common ancestor, an arboreal insectivore, a matter of great importance when considering the relationship of many of their parasites, as will be described in a later chapter. The evolution took place during the Cenozoic Era, or the Age of Mammals, which lasted about

70 million years (Table 1).* In the older epochs the mammals were mainly of archaic kinds, gradually giving place to the ancestors of the existing types. In the later epoch of the Tertiary there is considerable evidence of a gradual cooling of the North Temperate regions. This cooling culminated in the Pleistocene or Ice Age, in which portions of Europe and North America were covered several times with great glacial sheets of ice.

From the point of view of infectious disease, the geography of the Tertiary and Quaternary Periods is of considerable importance. America was cut off to a very large extent from the rest of the world, so that many of its mammals evolved separately. Furthermore, the north and south sections were largely divided from one another, resulting in even more separation. As a result, the early American prosimians and their descendants were removed by wide oceans from those of the Old World and the anthropoids that stemmed from them. In other words, monkeys evolved twice, once in the Old World, then separately and independently in South America. Fossil monkeys have been found in Middle to Late Cenozoic beds in South America, but none in North America. The importance of this is that the parasites of the two stocks are therefore likely to be different, so that the malaria of the one stock is not necessarily the same as that of the other, and yellow fever virus in monkeys could exist in Africa but not in South America until introduced by the activities of man.

Man is a product of the Ice Age or Pleistocene, which lasted about a million years. The geography of the world was altered markedly by the ice, for the ice sheets were one or two miles thick, like those of Greenland or the Antarctic today. The water that formed them came from the rain or snow which in turn originated in the oceans, and so much water was withdrawn in this fashion that the levels of oceans dropped by some hundreds of feet. During most of the million years of the Ice Age, the British Isles were part of the Continent, with the Thames being a tributary of the Rhine. Much of the Mediterranean was dry land and it was easy to cross to Africa. Ceylon was part of India; Australia was almost joined to Asia, except for

* Fossil magnetism and radioactive dating of rocks from eastern Australia and Tasmania have added new evidence that Australia was once much nearer the South Pole than it is today and has reached its present position only within the past 100 million years. In that short geological span, the Southern continent may have drifted as much as 3,000 miles with respect to North America and Europe at a rate approaching two inches a year. (Irving, E. and Evernden, J. F., quoted in *Scientific American,* June 1963, p. 73.)

See also "Continental Drift" by J. Tuzo Wilson. (*Scientific American,* April 1963.)

TABLE 1. TABLE OF GEOLOGIC PERIODS * (ROMER 1959)

Era (and duration)	Period	Estimated time since beginning of each period†	Life
Cenozoic (age of mammals; about 70 million years)	Quaternary	1	Modern species of mammals, extinction of large forms; dominance of man
	Tertiary	70	Rise of placental mammals and birds
Mesozoic (age of reptiles; lasted about 120 million years)	Cretaceous	120	Dominance of angiosperms commences; extinction of large reptiles and ammonites by end of period
	Jurassic	155	Reptiles dominant on land, sea, and in air; first birds; archaic mammals
	Triassic	190	First dinosaurs, turtles, ichthyosaurs, plesiosaurs; cycads and conifers dominant
Paleozoic (lasted about 360 million years)	Permian	215	Radiation of reptiles, which displace amphibians as dominant group; widespread glaciation
	Carboniferous	300	Fern and seed fern coal forests; sharks and crinoids abundant; radiation of amphibia; first reptiles
	Devonian	350	Age of fishes (mostly fresh-water); first trees and first amphibians
	Silurian	390	Invasion of the land by plants and arthropods; brachiopods; primitive jawless vertebrates
	Ordovician	480	Appearance of vertebrates (ostracoderms); brachiopods and cephalopods dominant
	Cambrian	550	Appearance of all invertebrate phyla and many classes; dominance of trilobites and brachiopods; diversified algae

* The older eras of earth history, before fossils became abundant, are omitted. The Carboniferous is generally subdivided into two periods, Mississippian (earlier) and Pennsylvanian (later). The time estimates are based on the rate of disintegration of radioactive materials found in a number of deposits.
† In millions of years.

a deep, narrow channel of water corresponding to Wallace's Line. This channel prevented most mammals except the bats and rats from crossing from Asia, so that the animals found on one side are largely different from those on the other, as pointed out by Wallace, the co-discoverer with Darwin, of natural selection. America was joined to Asia by dry land over what is now the Bering Straits. In Figure 2 are shown the contours of the sea bottom in this region today, where it will be seen that a drop in the level of the oceans of less than two hundred feet would convert the present-day channel to dry land. The ice sheets did not cover this land bridge, so that animals and man could and did cross from Asia.

With the melting of the ice, all this changed. Everywhere these land bridges were broken off. Furthermore, the weight of two miles of ice had pressed down the land beneath and pushed up the land beyond the ice face; so that with the release from this weight, a restoration took place with that land newly freed of ice springing back into place and the other sinking. All these changes resulted in animals being cut off on the isolated islands and continents. It was no longer easy or even possible for migrations from one continent to another to take place without the use of boats.

The higher apes first appeared in the later parts of the Tertiary and were confined to Africa and southeast Asia. The development of human characteristics almost certainly took place in Africa. In that continent in the past half century, an amazing collection of human and prehuman finds have been made there, leaving little doubt that this was the place of man's origin. Once it was thought that the great characteristic of man, his highly organized and developed brain, must have appeared first, but now it is obvious from the fossil remains that the first step was the acquisition of the erect mode of posture. The earliest men had small brains but walked upright. How many species of man evolved we do not yet know, but all others except our own died out.* There is only one species today.

* Efforts to define man probably go back to prehistoric times. One Greek described him as "a featherless biped," but Socrates ridiculed this attempt by spending the following night pulling the feathers off a chicken and producing his "man" in the morning. Queen Victoria, appalled by *The Origin of Species*, is said to have suggested to Sir Robert Owen, the greatest anatomist of his day, that he undertake the task, and obligingly he produced over 60 specific and definite differences between man and the other primates. Unfortunately, his fellow biologists soon showed that this was nonsense, but still the search goes on.

Homo has been described as *erectus, sapiens,* and the "toolmaker." However, a recent study by Miss Jane Morris-Goodall on chimpanzees in the wild state has shown that these primates can not only walk upright and think (which has been known for a long

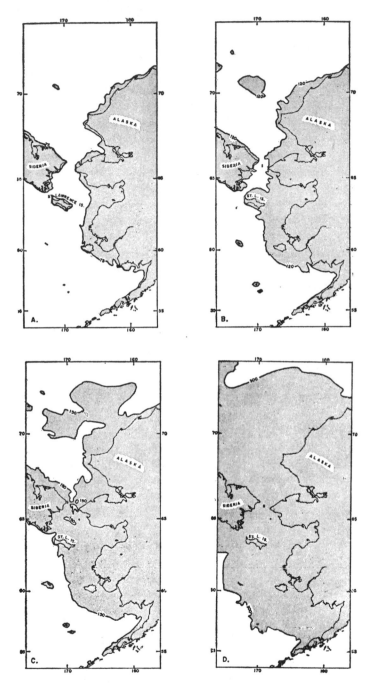

Figure 2. The probable outlines of the Alaskan and Siberian coasts when the sea level was (A) 75 feet, (B) 120 feet, (C) 150 feet, and (D) 300 feet below the present level. Shading indicates areas above sea level. [From David M. Hopkins (10)]

Of the extinct forms, the last to go was Neanderthal man who vanished about 30,000 years ago. Whether he was killed off by modern man or interbred with him is not known.

Modern man appeared only about 100,000 years ago.* Where he originated is not known, for the older theory that he evolved in Asia

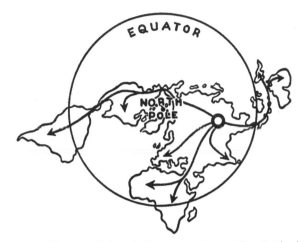

Figure 3. Dispersal of the principal races of man (after Matthew).

is now disputed by many who hold that he originated in Africa. The likely migration routes of this man are given in Figure 3, which was drawn in 1915 by Matthew on the basis of an Asian origin. However, even if this is incorrect and man was created in some African focus,

time), but also that they can use sticks as tools to catch termites for food. The latest definition by Dr. L. S. B. Leakey, therefore, is a combination of all these characters, so that a "true" man walks upright habitually and not only occasionally, holds his head straight, has a big brain and small face bones, and makes definite tools as a part of a recognizable culture (*Newsweek,* May 22, 1963, p. 98).

The truth is that in the evolutionary process of nature there never has been any sharp qualitative distinctions among the primates, only variations in degree. Man is a primate among fellow primates. His claim to specific rank depends upon his reproductive isolation from the others, but he comes from the same common stock. Never was there a certain point in time when a non-human primate pair gave birth to an infant that was the first human. Certain primates progressed from their original state to the one we now call "human," in a gradual fashion in the same way as the colors of the rainbow pass from one to the other.

* A book by Carleton Coons, recently published, challenges this concept of a unified origin of the races of man. Coons supports the older theories that the different races evolved in parallel from separate ancestors. Should this prove to be correct, it will alter the theories in this book only slightly, for of course even these separate ancestors come originally from a common stock. The only difference would be in talking in terms of millions of years instead of hundreds of thousands.

the main lines and ideas behind the chart of Matthew would still be correct except for the site of origin. Modern man reached Europe by 40,000 B.C. and replaced Neanderthal man who was already there. In America, the weapons of man are found intermingled with the bones of extinct animals such as an early bison and mammoths, so that he must have been there 20 or 30,000 years ago, having crossed the Bering land bridge. He had reached the tip of America by 7500 B.C. In Australia, old bones have been carbon dated back to about the same time. The aborigines there must have gone by boat, island hopping across the narrow strait while the sea level was still low. This would be long after the marsupials got there, but before the placentals arrived. The only placentals indigenous to Australia are man and his dog, the dingo, the bats which flew there, and the rats that presumably were carried there on floating debris. Man, of course, took his parasites with him.

With the ending of the Ice Age about 10 or 15,000 years ago, the sea levels rose and cut off these populations of people on to what are now the various continents. The only new invaders of America were those like the Eskimos who could cross the ice or paddle across the sea in boats. Australia remained remote, with only occasional visitors such as Malay fishermen, although there are suggestions in ancient writings that the Romans (who had trading stations in India) were vaguely aware that there existed animals like kangaroos. The islands of the Pacific were colonized by the Polynesian and other such sailors in the first millennium A.D. New Zealand was occupied also by these. During the Ice Age, North Africa enjoyed a heavy rainfall, and what is now the Sahara was a prairie-type land, heavily populated with many animals and the men who hunted them. Many rock paintings and carvings have been found in the Sahara, depicting animals like the hippopotamus in areas which now are completely without water. Some authorities think that as the Sahara dried up the people took refuge in the areas of permanent water such as the Nile valley.

As man wandered around the world, he would take many of his parasites with him. Those such as the louse, the pinworm, herpes virus, typhoid bacillus, and others that were closely attached to him would not have great trouble in traveling in this fashion. Others that required transmission by specific intermediate hosts would die out once the territory of the necessary intermediate hosts was left behind. In the home of man in Africa, for example, both early man and his precursors would be infected with schistosomes as are both man and the baboons of that continent today, but once man migrated into areas of the world where the snails that acted as intermediate hosts did not exist, then the infection would die out. In the same way, other infections such as trypanosomes and yellow fever virus would not survive a movement into areas where the necessary vectors were not present to transmit the pathogens. Malaria would be more likely to travel, since anopheline mosquitoes are found in many parts of the world. Here again, however, there would be limiting factors, mainly that of temperature. In regions where the temperature is too low for the development of the malaria parasite during the extrinsic cycle in the mosquito, the parasite would die out and man would be free of the infection. On the other hand, man arriving in a new territory might find the animals there carrying organisms to which he had not previously been exposed, but which were capable of infecting him. These might well invade his tissues successfully, and examples of this would be the Leishmania infections of rodents, both in South America and Asia, and the trypanosomal infections of armadillos in South America. In China and East Asia would be found Paragonimus infection with an intermediate host limited to that part of the world. In this fashion the basic pattern of infection of man would be established early in his days of migration. The development of more modern infections will be described later in this book.

THE PATHOGEN

In a later chapter it is theorized that all parasites and pathogens are descended from forms that originally were free living. From this come the questions as to why and how do free-living organisms become pathogenic for other creatures. Without doubt, in most instances the process is a slow one. Symbiosis or "living together" consists of a number of steps ranging from commensalism or "eating off the same table" and mutualism, which is an association without harm to either partner, to parasitism in which one partner lives at the expense of another, and finally to a state of pathogenicity in which the invader inflicts damage on its host to such an extent that the latter may be seriously injured or even killed. These matters are fully discussed in textbooks such as that of Caullery (11) and Topley and Wilson (4) and need no further discussion here, except for the question of pathogenicity. In the great majority of cases, a parasite does no noticeable harm to its host, except when present in overwhelming numbers; but in some instances, some adverse effect of its presence is accentuated to such a degree that it affects the well-being of its host and might even threaten the host's existence. This pathogenic effect has never been explained satisfactorily, so that we do not know why, for instance, many diphtheria organisms live peacefully and harmlessly in the human throat, while others develop a most deadly toxin that kills the host even in very weak dilutions. Nor do we know why the central nervous system should be invaded by so many viruses, bacteria, and protozoa whose normal biologic cycle includes periods in the respiratory, intestinal tracts, or blood, the latter being transmitted by vectors. So far as can be seen, none of these neurotropic characteristics has any essential role to play in the survival of the organism in question. However, the capacity of an organism to invade unusual environments like the central nervous system may have long-term survival values in that they provide a reserve of variation that is extremely useful when the environments change as they are bound to do sooner or later. This is mentioned later in the chapter on the concept of a species.

The definitions of pathogenicity and virulence used here are those proposed by Miles (12), in which pathogenicity is an attribute of a species, genus, or other such grouping of parasites, and virulence is reserved for the pathogenicity of a given stable line of microorganism. This is a very useful concept because of the great range of variation in the behavior of different strains of many animal viruses and bacteria. With this background, it is possible to define pathogenicity as the power to produce pathological effects in a host, and virulence as the evidence of pathogenicity derived from observation of the symptoms and signs of illness and death of the host (13).

Andrewes has suggested that in certain instances a parasite has something to be gained by being virulent to a certain degree, even though most accept Theobald Smith's dictum that there is a natural tendency of a host-parasite relationship toward a mutual tolerance which will permit a survival of both partners. One component of this tolerance is the increasing genetic resistance of the host to the parasite, a subject which is debated later under Theory 2. Andrewes points out that a respiratory tract organism has a better chance to spread if it causes the host to sneeze or cough, thus spreading it more widely in the population. Similarly, an intestinal organism that caused diarrhea will be excreted in larger quantities and thus will be more likely to find new susceptible hosts. On the other hand, many organisms of the respiratory and intestinal tracts create no such symptoms, but survive very nicely in spite of this.

Arbor viruses that are transmitted by arthropod vectors are dependent upon viremia, so that the vector can be infected and so transmit the infection. A high level and long-persisting viremia might therefore seem to be a great advantage to an arbor virus, but there is no great correlation between the severity of the disease and this viremia. Yellow fever persists in Africa where the monkeys have symptomless infections; in America the disease is often fatal to the monkeys. In these instances virulence is not noticeably associated with the capacity of the pathogen to survive.

Yet often when an organism has developed a high degree of pathogenicity for a certain host, there is a definite degree of correlation between the virulence of the various strains and the capacity of that pathogen to continue to exist. The most beautiful example of this has been shown by Fenner (14) to exist in the instance of the myxomatosis virus that was released deliberately among the rabbits of Australia. The most virulent strain was used and this killed off about 90 per cent of the rabbits of that time. However, the 10 per cent that escaped death were enough to rebuild the rabbit populations; and as time passed, not only have the rabbits become increasingly resistant to the virus, but the virus has lost a good deal of its virulence for the rabbits. This latter is explained on the grounds that a less virulent organism is more likely to survive, since the infected rabbit does not die so quickly and therefore more mosquitoes can feed on it and become capable of transmitting the virus. A more virulent strain has less chance of infecting the vector. Several times virulent strains have been released in Australia to maintain the killing effect, but always they have quickly vanished in competition with the existing semi-virulent ones. In England it is a different story, for there the vector is not the mosquito but the rabbit flea. Fleas do not usually desert their host while it still lives; only once it is dead do they search for another. The spread of the virus is therefore linked with the more increased virulence, for only when a flea leaves the rabbit that is dying of myxomatosis does the transmission take place. On the other hand, if too many rabbits die, the virus will have no hosts to infect and so die out itself also.

Andrewes' suggestion is therefore accepted that in many instances pathogenicity and a certain level of virulence can be of definite survival value to a parasite. The question now is whether a free-living organism can possess in its natural state the ability to be a pathogen when introduced for the first time to its host, or whether a long contact of host and potential pathogen is necessary for adaptation of one to the other and for the selection of pathogenic strains to proceed. For the great majority, presumably the latter is the normal course of events. An animal would pick up some organism in its environment that was preadapted to living within some cavity in its body; such an event would seem to be almost inevitable when it is considered that every animal is in contact with hosts of organisms every minute of its day, and that almost every cubic centimeter of the soil and water that surrounds it is teeming with millions of bacteria, protozoa, nematodes, mites, etc. Indeed it would be surprising if some sort of symbiosis did not take place, but of course there are limits to the number of organisms an animal's cavity can accommodate. An animal's body is obviously very satisfying as a source of food and shelter to many kinds of microorganisms. Once having become adapted to such matters as the higher temperature, the type of food available, and the various mechanisms of the host's defenses, the next step would be the invasion of the tissues. Again this is an almost inevitable step, for at all times the organisms in the body cavities are penetrating inside of the tissues. Every cut, every sore on the skin, every little weakness in the intestinal defenses gives access for all kinds of organisms to the tissues and body fluids and hence to the blood. Most of these will be dealt with by the body's defenses, but an occasional one will survive, and from this could spring a source of potential internal parasites and hence pathogens. This process will be discussed in more detail later in connection with Theory 1 and more specifically in the chapters on malaria, smallpox, tuberculosis, and the treponemotoses.

For the great majority of instances, this explanation seems adequate, but still unanswered is the question whether or not some free-living organisms can act immediately as pathogens. The most likely candidates for such a role are the fungi and acid-fast organisms which are known to be extremely common in the soil and some of which can give rise to disease. Ajello has listed a number of such organisms that are known to be actual or potential human pathogens (15). These include:

Absidia corymbifera
A. ramosa
Allescheria boydii
Aspergillus fumigatus

Candida albicans
C. guilliermondii
C. krusei
Coccidioides immitis

Cryptococcus neoformans
Epidermophyton floccosum
Histoplasma capsulatum
Microsporum gypseum
Nocarida asteroides
Phialophora jeanselmei
Phialophora pedrosoi

P. verrucosa
Rhizopus arrhizus
R. oryzae
Sporotrichum schenckii
Trichophyton mentagrophytes
T. rubrum

Table 2 lists the organisms he has isolated from soil.

TABLE 2. SOIL STUDY DATA (FROM AJELLO)

Locality	Sample (No.)	Allescheria boydii	Candida albicans	Cocci- dioides immitis	Crypto- coccus neofor- mans	Histo- plasma capsu- latum	Micro- sporum Gyseum
Tennessee *	710	15	1		5	67	30
Hawaii	100	1			1		23
Panama	100	1				1	36
Georgia †	79	2			2		13
Arizona ‡	48			1			
Michigan §	44						5
Nigeria	76				1		6
W. Virginia	16						2
Canada §	12						2
Maryland ‡	11				1		
Alabama	10				2		3
Venezuela ‡	5					4	
Peru ‡	4					1	
Totals	1,215	19	1	1	12	73	120
No. of soils tested for each fungus		1,141	1,141	48	1,141	1,141	439
Percentage positive		1.7	0.08	2.0	1.1	6.4	27.3

* Only 73 tested for *M. gypseum*.   ‡ Not tested for *M. gypseum*.
† Only 44 tested for *M. gypseum*.   § Not tested for *H. capsulatum*.

In human tuberculosis, most of the infections are due to the human or bovine species of *Mycobacterium,* but it is becoming increasingly obvious that many infections are due to other acid-fast organisms belonging to the same genus *Mycobacterium,* but of different species. These are now known as the anonymous or atypical acid-fast bacilli, and in the most recent classifications are subdivided into four main groups on the basis of pigment production with or without the action of light. Some of these bacilli seem to come from birds and be merely avian strains, but some are not yet linked to any animal infection and thus are candidates for the role of free-living organisms capable of causing human disease.

A decade or two ago, it seemed as though most of such soil pathogens were in fact free-living forms without any association with animals in the normal course of their existences. However, in some instances it has been shown that this is not really correct and that at some time or other, a period of time is spent in association with some animal. The most clear-cut of these associations is that of *Histoplasma capsulatum* and birds. *Histoplasma* has been recovered many times from soil, but several episodes of infections of man have been investigated which have shown that in the background there is some bird infection. That there is a substantial danger of acquiring histoplasmosis when cleaning out confined spaces contaminated with bird droppings has been long known, but a recent outbreak in Missouri in the open air was attributed to the droppings of starlings that roosted on trees. The soil under the trees was very heavily infected with *Histoplasma* (16).

Similarly, an acid-fast organism causing skin lesions and associated with swimming pools was given the name *M. balnei,* but now it is generally accepted that this is really the same as the fish pathogen *M. marinum.*

It may be that further studies will show that many or all of the so-called free-living pathogens have, in fact, some association with animals of one kind or another in their normal pattern of existence.

Very little is known of the ecology of organisms living in soil or water. Some are capable of metabolizing all their needs from very simple chemicals, while others apparently utilize products of other animals or plants either living or dead. The struggle of survival must be an intense one, judging by the number of organisms trying to occupy even the smallest ecological niche and apparently many of them have acquired weapons for defense in this struggle. One form of defense is the production of chemicals to kill or repel other organisms. As utilized in medicine, some of these go under the term of "antibiotics," the best known of these being penicillin produced by *Penicillium*. Perhaps many of the pathogenic effects of bacteria have arisen from some such mechanisms, being utilized by them and adapted according to their needs after a foothold has been obtained in the bodies of the future hosts. Perhaps the toxins of the diphtheria and botulism organisms arose in this fashion, although it is difficult to see how they benefit their producers.

THE ARTHROPOD VECTOR

Evolution of the Vectors

Modern thinking about the evolution of insects has been reviewed recently by Carpenter (17). It seems obvious that insects began life in an aqueous habitat and invaded the terrestrial world by some developmental step similar to the production of a water-tight skin by the reptiles. The earliest ones probably had no wings, although the opposite has also been suggested, that they arose from trilobites, the lateral lobes of which became wings. In support of the latter theory is the fact that there are records of winged insects (pterygota) from as far back as the Upper Carboniferous eras, but of wingless ones (apterygota) only as far back as the Triassic period. However, the reason for this may be that the wing is the only part of an insect that has a chance of surviving in geological strata, with the result that any wingless insect left little permanent impression for us to read today. The first records of insects are in the lowest Upper Carboniferous strata, and these had fully developed wings, though they could not fold them back over their bodies, being similar in that respect to dragonflies. The appearance of insects with folding wings followed later in the Upper Carboniferous period, and was a step of great importance in helping the insect to hide while at rest, especially when birds and flying reptiles appeared as predators.

The earlier insects had two sets of two wings, but later evolved so that the back pair were progressively reduced into non-functional vestiges. These Diptera, or two-winged insects, have provided many species that feed on blood and are therefore particularly suited for the transmission of pathogens from one animal to another. Included in this group are mosquitoes, tsetse flies, tabanids, as well as those that have completely lost their wings, the fleas and lice.

In considering the evolution of human infections, it is particularly important to know when the bloodsucking anthropods appeared in relation to man. It happens that vast numbers of fossil insects have been found in rocks and in amber—a fossil resin found especially in the Baltic area, where large forests of a particularly resinous type of pine tree once existed. Insects would fall into certain lakes and sink to the bottom, where they would be partially preserved in the mud, or else they might be trapped in the resin on a pine tree. In certain areas of Kansas and Colorado, a good day's search will produce about fifty fossil insects, while so many amber-preserved ones have been found that a museum in Germany had about a hundred thousand specimens.

Relying on the evidence of these fossils, it is often possible to say with certainty that a particular type existed in a certain era. In this way we know that mosquitoes, fleas, ticks, mites, tsetse flies, and many other potential vectors lived long before man appeared on earth. It is, therefore, possible that arthropod-transmitted infections appeared at a very early date—which does not necessarily mean that they actually did so. Table 3 gives a list of the fossil insects of present-day medical importance (18, 19), and it will be seen that all except lice have been dated back by fossil remains millions of years before the time of modern man.

The fleas, according to Ewing and Fox (20), are probably older and more primitive than Diptera. In support of this, they point out that the flea larva is more generalized and the adults lack the reduction and modification of the metathorax which is found on Diptera. Fleas probably developed from ancestors that still had functional metathoracic wings and were thus not true Diptera. The earliest known flea comes from Baltic amber, and is associated with those blue-grey clays that are usually assigned to the Oligocene, but may possibly have belonged to the Eocene. It was described by Dampf (21) and called *Palaeopsylla klebsiana* and there are twelve related species living today, most of them parasitic on shrews.

The fossil *Glossina* has been recovered from the Florissant shales near Pike's Peak, Colorado. This genus seems to have disappeared from the western hemisphere by the middle Tertiary (22), and at the present time is confined to Africa.

Many specimens of mosquitoes, closely resembling those of the *Culex pipiens* complex, have been recovered from the Baltic amber and demonstrate how little this species has altered in outward form in the intervening millions of years.

Since there are no records of lice before those found by Ewing (23) on the scalps of early American mummies, our conceptions of their descent and antiquity must be based on modern analogies. It was pointed out long ago by Kellogg (24) and Harrison (25) that the host distribution of permanent wingless parasites is governed more by the genetic relationships of their hosts than by any other ecological condition and that there is an intimate relationship between the phylogeny of the parasites and that of the hosts.

Webb (26) suggests that an ancient mallophagan ancestor arose

TABLE 3. EARLIEST RECORDS OF FOSSIL INSECTS

Period	Existing orders (after Carpenter 1952)	Some insects of medical importance, with number of specimens (after Schröder 1925 and Edwards 1932)	
Quaternary	Anoplura	*Culicidae*—5	*Culex* sp.—1
		Muscidae—34	
Tertiary	Enterotrophi	*Culicidae*—22	*Aedes* sp.—2
			Culex pipiens—6
			Culex sp.—10
	Isoptera	*Muscidae*—84	*Glossina*—4
	Embioptera	*Tabanidae*—2	*Pangoniinae*—2
	Siphonaptera	*Psychodidae*—23	*Phlebotominae*—19
	Lepidoptera	*Pulicidae*—3	*Palaeopsylla klebsiana*—3
		Reduviidae—1	
		Acarina—numerous	
		Trombidiidae	*Allothrombium*—1
			Dermacentor—1
Cretaceous		*Culicidae*—1	
Jurassic	Thysanura	*Culicidae*—1	*Culex* sp.—1
	Dermaptera	*Psychodidae*—3	
	Trichoptera		
	Diptera		
	Hymenoptera		
Triassic	Orthoptera		
Permian	Plecoptera		
	Thysanoptera		
	Coleoptera		
	Odonata		
	Ephemeroptera		
	Meroptera		
	Strepsiptera		
	Neuroptera		
	Corrodentia		
	Hemiptera		
Carboniferous	Orthoptera	*Blattidae*	
Devonian	Collembola	*Acarina*	

from Psocida, some of which are common in bark, detritus, and birds' nests. When these mallophagans migrated to mammals, new lines would arise, the lice of marsupials and guinea pigs coming from Amblycera, and Trichodectidae and Siphunculata being derived from the same Ischnoceran ancestor. The most primitive mammalian form

found was that of a tree-shrew parasite, which was strongly remi-
niscent of the common chicken parasite, *Eomenacanthus straminius,*
thus suggesting a very early origin for the Siphunculata. The origin
of mammalian lice may well have been in the migration of a primitive
Ischnoceran parasite from a bird to a primitive arboreal insect-eater,
so that there were undoubtedly lice on the primates long before
man put in his appearance. Lice of the genus *Pediculus* are confined
to the Order Primates (Ewing).

The Environment

The environment is never static; always it is changing—sometimes
quickly and sometimes slowly—and with it change the creatures
living within its limits. The curious thing is that man himself, who
to a large extent shapes his own environment (27), will no doubt in
turn be altered by his own creation. A full work on the changing
world and its effects on the infections of man and his ancestors would
occupy several books. All that can be done here is to note some of
the major developments in the past tens of thousands of years that
have influenced the patterns of these infections. No mention will
be made of the geographic variations, for those dealing with the
alterations in the shapes of land masses will be referred to in the
appropriate places in later chapters; nor of temperature fluctuations, although it is obvious that cold spells in the world's history
must have had marked effects upon the distributions of insect vectors,
hosts, and parasites like that of malaria which have a temperature
requirement. The emphasis here will be on man of the last hundred
millennia—man the tool maker, the hunter, the nomad with his
herds, the farmer, the sailor, the industrial worker, and today's man,
speeding at several times the speed of sound. All these men have
had infectious diseases, but these have varied from time to time and
place to place. To understand those infections we have with us today,
and to try to predict what we may have tomorrow, we must first study
how, why, and when they altered in the past in response to changes
in the environment. For this purpose, we must appreciate the variations in those environments.

Man the Hunter

In the very early days primitive man lived like a wild animal
among other wild animals, but by the time modern man developed,

fire and the use of primitive tools and weapons had already been discovered, so that he was a hunter instead of the hunted. Improved techniques and better food supplies led to greater populations, but even so the actual numbers remained small. People lived in widely scattered bands, the concentration in any one area depending on the amount of food available—in order to support himself by hunting, the forest-dwelling American Indian was said to require 5 square miles of territory. In Australia today, the area required per aborigine is huge, with a marked inverse correlation with rainfall (28). In some favorable locations, communities of hunters were established and permanent fishing villages were set up along the banks of rivers or lakes where fish were easy to catch, but in no case was there a really heavy concentration of people (29).

The era of hunting reached its climax toward the end of the Ice Age. Up to that time vast herds of animals, such as deer, horses, wild cattle, as well as mammoths and cave bears, roamed Europe, and a more tropical variety ranged over the whole of Africa. In North America, an extinct form of buffalo and mammoth was very numerous and many human artifacts have been found in association with their bones (30). In most parts of the world there was plenty to hunt and much to eat. We know that this was the case in Europe because of evidence such as the wonderful paintings in the caves of southern France and northern Spain, painted about 15,000 years ago and just as fresh as when first executed, and all about the animals that were hunted. In Bohemia, man used to trap the mammoths in pits as they came on migration down certain valleys and as many as a thousand skeletons of these mammoths have been found in one midden heap. But in spite of this apparent abundance of food, man was still a rare animal, living in small groups, limited by the food factor—the feast of one day would be followed by several of famine. For example, the Indians following the buffalo had no horses, for horses were not present until introduced by the Spaniards. They had to move with the herds, hanging on the outskirts in the hopes of picking off stragglers or stampeding part of the herd over a cliff. When a big hunt was successful, everyone gorged down as much meat as possible, for there was no good way of preserving the remainder. Two weeks later the tribe might be starving. Incidentally, Regina, Saskatchewan, was originally called "Pile o' Bones" after one such successful buffalo hunt. Some, like the Fort Ancient Indians in Ohio, settled by a stream beside a big bed of mussels and lived on these together with deer and smaller animals they could trap and fruit they could collect. In time they learned to grow squash. But the number of people that can be supported in an area in this fashion is quite limited. Large towns cannot be supported on a hunting economy. If the people of New York had to eat only those animals they could kill hunting, all the modern problems of obesity and overeating would soon disappear from that city.

Man the hunter, traveling from place to place as do the bushmen of the Congo, the aborigines of Australia, the Hadza hunters of Tanganyika today, was not only a fairly rare creature but also a lonely one. His family groups or tribes were small and isolated, with little contact with one another except for ceremonial meetings and the occasional trader. However, many races, like the Australian aborigines, mated only with women from outside the tribe, so that genetically and parasitically there was a 50 per cent exchange every generation between tribes within the bounds of such cultural patterns.

Trade did exist to some limited extent between purely hunting communities. It is well known that during the Stone Age men would travel long distances to obtain pieces of flint for tools, if there were none in the places where they lived; and furthermore, certain workers specialized in making the flint tools. At Brandon in Suffolk, England, are big deposits of flint of good quality; for many thousands of years specialists have worked this material and other people have come long distances to obtain the tools they made. Even today, or at least twenty years ago, when I was last in that area, there were four or five men, the flintknappers of Brandon, still carrying on the unbroken tradition of many thousands of years, only now they make flints for flintlock guns, not axes and knives. In North America, the traveling salesmen of about 800 years ago were the Hopewell Indians. Traveling on foot or by canoe, they covered the whole of the area from the Atlantic to the Rockies, exchanging the large shells of the Bay of Mexico for the copper from the Great Lakes or the obsidian for sacrificial knives from the deposits in Wyoming (31). In paleolithic times in Europe, the cave dwellers who painted the pictures on the walls of caves obviously traded with people hundreds of miles away.

It is surprising, in fact, to discover how fast man can travel using only his own legs. When in West Africa, I was continually coming across long-legged Africans, walking swiftly along the road leading north from Kumasi, and, on inquiring, was told that these were people who carried dried fish from the Niger, many hundreds of miles from the north to Kumasi. At Kumasi they sold the fish and bought a load of kola nuts to take back to the Niger. One day I happened to notice a small group setting off in the twilight of the early morning, as I was leaving in my lorry for a village 30 miles away. By noon they had reached this village, so I stopped them with the offer of food. Through an interpreter they said they were sleeping the night 20 miles farther on. They apparently covered this distance with their loads every day and must have averaged 40 or 50 miles a day. In South America, before the Spaniards, there were no horses. The Incas set up a system of runners, where each runner ran at top speed for one mile and then handed on his message to the next runner. The distance involved was about 600 miles and messages were carried faster by this means than by the equivalent pony express in North America. Chaka, King of the Zulus, made his soldiers discard their sandals so that their feet could be hardened for faster running. A Zulu impi could cover 50 miles in one night (32).

Trading among the Eskimos before the white man had noticeably altered their civilization has been described by Petroff (1879) in his account of an Eskimo day: "Evening is approaching, the people are scattering about the village, when away in the distance on the ice of the river two sleds appear in sight, and children playing on the river bank are the first to discover them; but no particular attention is paid to the incident. The travellers approach and put up at one of the dwellings; it is a family consisting of a man, a woman, a grown-up daughter and a small boy. Nobody meets them but the new arrivals seem perfectly at home, tie their dogs to the posts of the storehouse, discharge their lot of provisions or utensils, and place the sleds on top of the roof. The women and boy then enter the house while the man proceeds to the Kashga, which he enters without any solicitations; in fact words of greeting are missing in the vocabulary of this people. . . . The stranger has not come to see anybody in particular, but wishes to dispose of some goods in exchange for other articles he needs. . . . He brings into the Kashga all he wishes to barter declaring at the same time that for such an article he wishes to exchange such other commodity. . . . Here comes a man who purchased something of the stranger a year or two previously, but ruing the bargain returns the article saying simply 'This does not suit me.' The other picks it up and returns without any remonstrance anything he has in his possession of equal value with the original price" (33).

Much of the trading in ancient times was by means of "Silent Barter." Two groups of people, wishing to exchange goods but neither trusting the other, would in turn lay their goods side by side on the ground, then retreat to allow the other to approach. Additions or subtractions to the piles of goods would be made until agreement was reached, and then the exchange would be made without either party ever coming into contact with the other. Such a system was widespread until modern times, and indeed was the first method of trading employed by Europeans on the West African coast. The Portuguese improved on this form of trading by erecting a fort on the beach before the Africans could attack them. The fort, which still stands at Elmina, Ghana, was prefabricated in Portugal about A.D. 1450, the stones numbered and carried to Africa on numerous ships, and a landing made. A tower was hastily built in one day before the local tribes had time to gather a fighting force. Trading by "Silent Barter" is a great impediment to the spread of infectious diseases.

Allowing for all these facts, travel in the hunting era was not an everyday event, and much of the barter must have been a slow business. Undoubtedly, infections could travel along the trade routes, but it would be a slow and chancy business compared with what developed once agriculture provided quantities of goods for trade, specialized traders, and better means of transport.

Hunting man had few animals living as parasites or commensals in his ecological niche as does man today, although he lived closely to those he hunted. Beyond his dog, no animal accompanied him on his travels. All the remainder, the horse, cow, and goat, the chicken, sparrow and pigeon, the mosquitoes specializing on his blood, the rat and mouse, all of these could only come and live with him when he settled down or deliberately trained some of them to travel in herds for his own convenience. This happened only after the Ice Age had gone, and the herds of big animals had disappeared from Europe, the Sahara and, except for the buffalo, from the plains of North America. It was at this point that man made the biggest change in his life since he had learned to stand upright. He discovered the secrets of agriculture and how to domesticate animals.

Man the Farmer

Man the hunter always lived a very precarious existence, having a feast one day and a famine a short time after; his big difficulty was that he could not store food to tide him over a period of scarcity. The discovery of a technique whereby he could deliberately create food in a quantity adequate enough and of a kind that could be stored had a tremendous effect on the whole world. No longer did surplus children have to be killed at birth, nor old people put out to die when no longer able to provide or look after themselves. There was food for all, and the world population increased in leaps and bounds. Large cities appeared and civilization in its modern sense became possible.

The actual discovery that certain plants and fruits could be cultivated was made separately in several parts of the world. Wheat seems to have been grown first in the drier uplands of what is now Turkey. Rice seems to have originated farther east in Asia. From Central and South America came maize, squash, and the potato. Probably the earliest of these events occurred about 5 or 6,000 years before Christ. The sequence of events is well demonstrated by the excavations at Jericho in the Jordan Valley. The site was obviously a desirable one because of the permanent spring of water, the Ain es Sultan, and originally Mesolithic hunters settled there and built a sanctuary. The date of their occupation has been fixed at 7800 B.C. by means of carbon dating, and the site they chose has had a continuous sequence of occupation ever since.

A thousand or so years later, agriculture was being practiced and a permanent township had been erected which lasted until biblical times. The area is still heavily farmed, using irrigation water from the original spring, and in 1946, when I was last there, a small town was located near the ancient site. By 4000 B.C. there were cities in Iraq with populations of 400,000 people, and thriving civilizations in China, the valley of the Indus, and the Nile, all supported by the food grown from the practice of agriculture.

So far as infectious disease was concerned, it was not only the increase in population that was important, but also the fact that commerce, with its potential for spread of pathogens, now developed on a fairly large scale. With an agricultural economy, not everyone had to produce food. There was enough to support not only the farmers and their families, but also a class of artisans, priests, traders, teachers, and other skilled and professional classes. Goods of all kinds were produced, and the demand for more of these and of an increasingly varied type stimulated trade between communities.

The most important means of transport apart from a man's legs was the boat. A hollow log was adequate for crossing a river, but to transport large loads on open water, something more was needed. Plank boats were made in Egypt probably during the fourth millen-

nium B.C. The earliest actual record of a sailing boat is a clay toy
from Erido in Mesopotamia dated 3500 B.C. By the time of the
Romans there were freighters up to 1,200 tons and as big as the Con-
stitution. In the time of Caligula, the largest ship then made carried
1,300 tons of lentils from Cairo to Rome, while another brought
from Egypt the obelisk which now stands in front of St. Peters in
Rome and which weighs 500 tons and is 130 feet high (34). With
ships like these, communication between the great centers of civilization was a practical matter. The Romans had a series of trading
posts in India; the Pharaoh Neccho sent Phoenician explorers around
Africa and they made the trip in three years. The Chinese traded
with all southeast Asia. However, the boats at first were very primitive
and avoided the open sea. One of the most difficult coasts was along
the southern edge of Persia, a most dry and desolate land with very
poor harbors, as Alexander the Great found on his march back from
India. However, the land there is rising and present day conditions are not necessarily those of previous times. Some thousands
of years ago it was much easier to travel along the coast, as shown
by the excavations at Sutkagen-dor on the Makran Coast. During
the days of the great city of Harappa in the Indus valley, Sutkagen-
dor must have been a seaport on a wide estuary, but now it is on
dry and desert land thirty miles from the nearest sea. Probably
there was substantial traffic between Harappa and the civilization
in Mesopotamia (35). About the time of Christ, a sailor discovered
the secret of the monsoons and that the trip from Africa to India,
directly across the Indian Ocean, could be made at the proper seasons
in three weeks, instead of six months by hugging the coast. The
Romans erected a monument at the entrance to the Red Sea to honor
the discoverer (34).

Man the Sailor

Before Christ, the world was divided into communities that had
little or no real contact with one another, except perhaps for the
kind described above. The largest concentrations of people were
found in Central America, the Mediterranean, the Nile valley, Iraq,
India, and China and southeast Asia. Some of these were entirely
isolated and the others were linked only by slow and intermittent
caravans and occasional ships. The people of lands such as southern
and central Africa, Australia, and the Arctic lived by themselves, not
knowing that the others existed. The islands of the Pacific had not

yet been colonized. This state of affairs continued so long as man had no boats capable of encountering the open sea, nor means of navigation. Until these difficulties were overcome, and close contact made between the people, there could be little spread of infection from one to the other. A man in America may have one kind of pathogen, and others in Africa or Australia could have other kinds and there was no means by which there could be an interchange. The invention of the ocean-going ship, the discovery of the compass, and the use of the stars for navigation changed all that. In the first millennium after Christ, there were Polynesian sailors crossing the Pacific in all directions, Malays fishing off the coasts of Australia, Vikings exploring the North Atlantic and reaching out to America. Arab sailors were colonizing East Africa and trading all over the Indian Ocean. In the second millennium came the discovery and colonizing of all inhabitable land in all parts of the world. Interchange of animals, both wild and domestic, of vectors and parasites, now took place on an increasing scale, in the new rats invading Europe, plague appearing in the form of the Black Death, yellow fever, smallpox, measles, and possibly malaria being imported into America. Cholera, in the nineteenth century, spread over the world from Bengal, and in 1918 influenza swept to the most remote communities on all continents.

Traders brought filariasis from the South Seas to Egypt. Slaves brought hookworms and schistosomes from Africa to America. Today this process is being accentuated so that approximately 70,000 people in New York, 2,000 in Chicago, and 1,500 in Philadelphia are infected with the blood fluke *S. mansoni* (36).

The Industrial Revolution

This began in England in the eighteenth century and rapidly spread over Europe and hence to the world in general. In what are now termed the "emerging countries," the full impact of the revolution is just arriving. Industry differs from arts and crafts in that machines are used to increase the output capacity of one man. Goods of all kinds can be produced cheaply and in large quantities. At first sight, this would seem to lead to a great increase in wealth for the population, but unfortunately the most immediate result seems to be the concentration of large numbers of peoples within areas around the industries, under conditions of overcrowding and poor hygiene. The slums of England in the first half of the nineteenth century were appallingly bad, and their counterparts are being created rapidly in too many countries in Africa and Asia today. Ignorance, poverty, overcrowding, dirt, starvation, these seem to be the earliest products of most industrial revolutions, and in their train comes a host of infectious diseases. Smallpox, cholera, typhus, typhoid, dysentery, measles, tuberculosis, and diphtheria were commonplace in Europe in the nineteenth century, together with scarlet fever, that great killer of its time. This latter never gained a foothold in the tropics and for some reason, which has never been properly explained, changed to a very mild disease in the twentieth century.

The opinion is expressed later that perhaps cholera evolved into its pandemic form as the result of the creation of the great insanitary city of Calcutta.

The Jet Age

Travelers can now journey from one continent to another at almost the speed of sound. Of course the pathogens carried by the passengers can do likewise. So far as infectious diseases are concerned, this is the "One World" of Wendell Willkie. The first effect of this is to require an urgent revision of our quarantine practices, for many of them are already out of date. Since it is possible for a man to travel from one spot on the globe to almost any other within the space of the incubation period of most pathogens, there are no good means of detecting infected persons. A man infected with cholera could be in Calcutta one day and in two days be in New York and yet appear quite healthy on arrival. The vaccination against cholera is no guarantee of solid protection against the disease. In the winter of 1961–62, several outbreaks of smallpox occurred in Europe, being imported from Pakistan and Africa. In the past, Europe had been protected not so much by quarantine measures as by the fact that it took several weeks by ship to travel there from Asia and Africa, and any cases of smallpox became obvious in that time. The jet plane has altered all of that.

The Domestication of Animals

The domestication of animals played two very important roles in influencing the infections of man. First, by providing a substantial and steady source of food, it led to a marked increase in population and hence to the appearance of crowd infections; and second, the animals themselves were almost certainly the source of many of the pathogens that were transferred to man and in time became adapted to him, becoming specifically human infections. This is discussed in more detail later, this section being confined to the actual domestication itself.

Hunting man had only one animal, the dog. This animal had apparently been associated with him for a long time and presumably was of use to him in the actual hunting.

The strongest argument in favor of the Australian aborigine crossing to that continent by boat is that the only other placental on the continent (apart from bats and rats) is his dog, the dingo. It could cross in his boat over the water that stopped other placentals. Several authorities have argued that the hunter tamed no other animal, and cite the examples of such people and animals as the Indians and the buffalo, the Australian aborigines and the marsupials, or the bushman with the African fauna, such as the eland; none of these people have any domesticated animals, although the animals they hunted are easily tamed. "The cultural thesis which has been most widely accepted is that which asserts that cattle, probably the first of the great herd animals to be domesticated were originally domesticated in western Asia. This thesis further argues that the domesticators of cattle were sedentary farmers rather than nomadic hunters, that domestication was deliberately undertaken and not haphazard, and that the motive was religious" (37). Some animals such as the dog and wild pig may have sought out man by scavenging around his camp, and gradually man assumed the leadership in the association. Something of this sort can be seen today in the national parks, where the bears come close to the camps at night looking for something to eat; some have so lost the fear of man that they sit by the roadside begging, and even push their snouts through the car windows.

In the woods of Canada, the Canada jay or whisky jack simply haunts the camps in the most friendly fashion and with even the least encouragement moves in beside the campers. Even today piglets and dog pups are nursed by woman in primitive societies. But the domestication of the larger herbivores cannot be explained along these lines.

"Esuard Hahn has postulated that the motive for capturing horned animals, such as the goat and sheep and above all the wild cattle, was the shape of their horns which resembled the crescent moon. The mother goddess was worshiped over an immense area of the ancient world and she was closely linked with the moon, so that an animal like a cow would be likely to be caught for sacrificial purposes. Studies in prehistoric and early historic religion have shown that the bovine was really regarded as an epiphany of the goddess or her consort and was slain in the ritual re-enactment of the myth of her death. The sequence of events would be as follows: the captured animals would be kept in corrals waiting sacrifice, where they would be protected from predators and able to breed. The young—born under captivity—would be more tractable than their parents and so capable of being used in a wider range of rituals which would include the first harnessing, and indeed the first known harnessing of cattle was to sleighs or wagons in religious processions. Mesopotamian frescos show priests using cattle for plowing and performing other tasks of husbandry, sacrificing them, or using them in processions. Castration of the bull which led to one of the most significant of agricultural developments, the ox, had also a religious origin, being probably modeled on the human ritual castration that re-enacted the fate of the diety in certain cults" (37). The bull dancing in Minoan Crete was probably religious in origin, and its modern equivalent in Spain today, which ends with the death of the bull, was probably similarly motivated in the beginning.

Devising a harness for a bull to be used in traction is not an easy matter, and the earliest ones depicted from ancient times are of very inefficient types, presumably derived from the restraints used in processions. Ropes were tied to the horns or to a stick fashioned between the horns, which, of course, would be of some use but not very much. The neck yoke was not known until about 1600 B.C. in Egypt. In spite of this, sleds and wagons or pictures of them have been found in many parts of Mesopotamia by the third millennium B.C. and must have been in use by the fourth.

Of the other animals, the horse first comes into history with the Hittites, or rather the donkey which was harnessed to chariots. The horse was derived from the tarpan of Asia. There are still a few specimens of the wild horse, Prjevalsky's horse, left in zoos today, and the wild ass still exists in Asia. The cat came from Egypt where it was an epiphany of the goddess Bast. Huge numbers of mummified cats have been found near Bubastis and these show it was descended from the Libyan wild cat. The name Tabby is of Egyptian origin; the Semitic post-biblical term for a cat was the "swaddled," referring to the mummification; and it is likely that the word cat itself may be ultimately derived from the old Semitic word for cotton (37).

The pigeon is descended from the wild rock dove. The chicken is from the East and comes from the jungle wild fowl; the smaller variety, the bantam, is named for the town of that name in Indonesia. The rabbit came from Spain, where the wild kind was trapped and kept in enclosures for hunting. The Romans adopted the sport and introduced it to the rest of Europe. The British took the rabbit to Australia. The pig's ancestors were descended from the wild boar: the fact that so many people regard it as unclean, or rather not to be eaten, suggests that originally it was a sacred animal just as is the cow in India today. In America, the Incas had domesticated the llama and also kept herds of vicunas. Animals like sheep and goats are obviously derived from the similar wild stock.

Mosquitoes like *Anopheles gambiae* and *Aedes aegypti* are now closely linked to man's ecology, but the wild forest types that presumably gave rise to these strains still exist in the forest of Africa.

From the point of view of infectious disease, a most significant event was the spread of the rat. The first rat to arrive in Europe was the black house or ship rat, and the first time in history this is clearly recorded is by Giraldus Cambiensis (1147–1223). Authorities agree that it came from the East, and according to de l'Isle (38), it was a wild rodent of Arabia that became parasitic on man about the seventh century and spread in the ships of the Crusaders. By the thirteenth century it had become a pest all over Europe, and the groundwork had been laid for great medieval epidemics of plague like the Black Death of the fourteenth century. Zinsser suggests that human louse-borne typhus in epidemic form arose from flea-borne rat typhus during the great wars in Central Europe in the fifteenth century, when conditions were favorable for the evolution of an infection of this type. If so, then all the millions of deaths from epidemic typhus can be laid at the feet of the black rat (39).

Later, he was pushed aside by a more ferocious invader from Mongolia, the brown rat, which appeared in Europe sometime in the eighteenth century. It migrated overland, overcoming all the natural obstacles in its way—Pallas records in his Zoögraphica Rosso Asiatica (1831) that in 1727 great masses of these rats swam the Volga after an earthquake. Their subsequent spread over the world was undoubtedly by ship, and they reached England in 1728, America in 1775. At the present time they are world-wide in distribution and carry many infectious diseases to man, including plague, typhus, trichinosis, rat-bite fever, and leptospirosis.

REFERENCES

1. HUXLEY, J. S.: *Evolution: A Modern Synthesis*. Harper & Bros., New York, 1942.
2. ROMER, A. S.: *The Vertebrate Story*. 4th Ed. Univ. of Chicago Press, Chicago, 1959.
3. DARWIN C.: *The Origin of Species*. 6th Ed. John Murray, London, 1906.
4. TOPLEY AND WILSON: *Principles of Bacteriology and Immunity*. 4th ed. Williams & Wilkins, Baltimore, 1955.
5. MAYR, E.: *Systematics and the Origin of Species*. Columbia Univ. Press, New York, 1942.
6. MILLER, S. L.: A production of amino acids under possible primitive earth conditions. Science, 1953, **117**: 528.
7. LORBSACK, T.: *Our Atmosphere*. Pantheon, New York, 1959.
8. OPARIN, A. I.: *The Origin of Life on Earth*. 3rd Rev. Academic Press, New York, 1957.
9. LAIDLAW, P. P.: *Virus and Virus Diseases*. Cambridge Univ. Press, Cambridge, 1938.
10. HOPKINS, D. M.: Cenozoic history of the Behring land bridge. Science, 1959, **129**: 1519–28.
11. CAULLERY, M.: *Parasitism and Symbiosis*. Sidgwick & Jackson, Ltd., London, 1952.
12. MILES, A. A.: quoted by Stuart-Harris C. H. in *Virus, Virulence and Pathogenicity*. Little, Brown & Co., Boston, 1960.
13. ANDREWES, C. H.: The effect on virulence of changes in parasite and host in *Virus, Virulence and Pathogenicity*. Little, Brown & Co., Boston, 1960.
14. FENNER, F.: Myxomatosis. Brit. Med. Bull., 1959, **15**: 240–45.
15. AJELLO, L.: The soil as a natural reservoir for human pathogenic fungi. Science, 1956, **123**: 876–78.
16. FURCOLOW, M. L.: Airborne histoplasmosis. Bact. Rev., 1961, **25**: 301–9.
17. CARPENTER, F. M.: The geological history and evolution of insects. Amer. Scientist, 1953, **41**: 256–70.
18. SCHRODER, F.: *Handbuch der Entomologie*. **3,** Gustav Fischer, Jena, 1925.
19. EDWARDES, F. W.: Oligocene mosquitoes in the British Museum. Quart. J. Geol. Soc., 1923, **79**: 139–55. Also in Culicidae section, Coytsmans *Genera Insectorum*, 1932.
20. EWING AND FOX, I.: *Fleas of North America*. Charles C Thomas, Baltimore, 1943.
21. DAMPF A.: Palaeopsylla klebsiana. Konisberg Schr. physik Ges., 1910, **51**: 248–59.
22. COCKERILL, T. D. A.: Fossil insects from Florissant. Colo. Bull. Amer. Mus. Nat. Hist., 1908, **24**: 65–66.
23. EWING, H. E.: *A Manual of External Parasites*. Charles C Thomas, Baltimore, 1929.
24. KELLOGG, V. L.: Distribution and species forming of Ectoparasites. Amer. Naturalist, 1913, **47**: 129–58.
25. HARRISON, L.: The Mallophaga as a possible clue to bird phylogeny. Aust. Zool., 1914, **1**: 7–11.
26. WEBB, J. E.: Phylogenetic relationships of the anoplura. Proc. Zool. Soc., London, 1946, **116**: 49–119.
27. CHILDE, G. V.: *Man Makes Himself*. A Mentor Book, New America Library, 1951.
28. TINSDALE, N. B.: Distribution of Australian aboriginal tribes. Trans. Roy. Soc. South Australia, 1940, **64**: 140–231.
29. BIRDSELL, J. B.: Population structure in generalized hunting populations. Evolution, 1958, **12**: 189–205.
30. WORMINGTON, H. M.: *Ancient Man in North America*. Denver Mus. Nat. Hist., 1957.

31. From an exhibit in the Field Museum, Chicago.
32. RITTER, E. A.: *Chaka Zulu*. Putnam, New York, 1957.
33. PETROFF, 1879. Quoted by Anderson H. D. and Eels, W. C.: *Alaska Natives*. Stanford Univ. Press, Stanford, 1935.
34. CASSON, L.: *Ancient Mariners*. Macmillan, New York, 1959.
35. DALES, G. F.: Harappan outposts on the Makran Coast. Antiquity, 1962, **36:** 86–92.
36. CHANDLER, A. C. AND READ, C. P.: *An Introduction to Parasitology*. John Wiley & Son, New York, 1961.
37. ISAAC, E.: On the domestication of cattle. Science, 1962, **137:** 195–204.
38. HIRST, F. L.: *The Conquest of Plague*. Clarendon Press, Oxford, 1953.
39. ZINSSER, H.: *Rats, Lice and History*. Little, Brown & Co., Boston, 1935.

CHAPTER 3

Paleoepidemiology

EPIDEMIOLOGY IN MODERN TIMES has not been defined to the satisfaction of all those using the term. Originally, it was applied to the study of epidemics, as is obvious from the name itself, but when it was found that epidemics could not be understood without reference to the occurrence of infections between epidemic periods, the term came to be applied to the study of infections at all times. The practitioners of this form of epidemiology in the course of their inquiries invented various procedures and statistical techniques, and some of these were found to be of value and general application in many other disciplines. This extension of epidemiologic techniques was hastened by the dramatic disappearance from the Western world of the major killing infections of the last century such as smallpox, cholera, yellow fever, typhus, etc., which of necessity has forced the schools of public health to look for new non-infectious fields to conquer. However, the term epidemiology in these "non-infectious" disciplines is largely limited to the statistical techniques, which is only one section of the total as applied to infectious diseases. In its original form it had a much wider meaning, and included such matters as diagnosis of disease, microbiology, the biology of insect vectors, laboratory techniques, geography, climate, population studies, migrations of peoples, and trade routes; it is still used in this sense by the students of infectious diseases. Much of the work of Hippocrates can be classed as epidemiology in its original meaning.

One feels that practitioners of the statistical techniques in fields other than those of infectious disease should invent a new name for their discipline instead of utilizing a term that already has been appropriated for another, and is neither descriptive nor properly applicable to their own. The use of terms such as the "epidemiology" of mental disease or road accidents is to be deplored.

Most of the papers in this book are considered to be epidemiologic in nature, and yet in the whole work, the use made of statistical analysis is absolutely minimal and simple to the point of being not much more than plain common sense. Epidemiology in this sense is a section of biology dealing with the interplay of man and his parasites within the ecologic niches of both. That is the way in which the term is used in this work.

With epidemiology in general defined as the study of the ecology of infectious diseases, paleoepidemiology is that of infectious diseases before modern times. It refers particularly to the maintenance and spread of infections in the days and eras of mankind prior to the maintenance of accurate records of disease, going back thousands of millions of years to the origin of life. Neoepidemiology is that of the last two or three hundred years, and especially the last fifty years, during which time precise identification of organisms, insect vectors, intermediate hosts, animal reservoirs, and all the techniques of modern science have permitted a high level of understanding of the ecology of infections. By definition, therefore, paleoepidemiology is as yet an imprecise science, in which facts are few and speculation is dominant.

Paleoepidemiology can be divided into two components, the vertical and horizontal transmission of infections. Horizontal spread is that form of epidemiology normally studied; a pathogen is transmitted from one community to another within the human race, as for example the pandemic of Asian flu in 1957 that traversed the world in a brief time, or from an animal source to a human population as occurs in the zoonoses. Such processes could have happened at any time in the human population during the million years of man's separate existence on earth, or in the hundreds of millions of years during the evolution of his predecessors. Vertical spread is the maintenance and transmission of a parasite within a group, perhaps a small one, over vast periods of time. In that time, the host groups will sooner or later split into separate groups, each carrying the parasite, and these isolated units will begin to vary from one another to the extent that new species will evolve. All will still carry the parasite, so that eventually the situation will arise in which a number of species removed in one way or another from one another will be parasitized by a common organism. This is a well-known phenomenon in biology and is expressed in the saying that related hosts have related parasites. It is described in more detail in the chapter dealing with evolution. These two means of transmission are of course closely linked with one another, for at any time a parasite that is being maintained vertically can spread to another animal that moves into the ecology of its permanent host, as happens in the zoonoses, where an animal infection spreads to a human; on the other hand, such an accidental infection might find conditions in the new host suitable for permanent existence there, and in time, the repeated transmission within the new population might lead to the selection of a new strain of parasite. In large scale epidemics of the arthropod transmitted infections of plague and Q fever, direct respiratory spread from man to man often occurs, and if this were to be continued for several years, then new strains of *Pasteurella* and *Rickettsia* might well appear. Later it will be theorized that this was the process by which the pox viruses evolved from animals in man's ecology; at first, there would be vertical transmission within a single animal group for millions of years, with horizontal spread a few thousand years ago to the newly evolved domestic animals living with the human group, and subsequent vertical transmission within these domestic animals and man, and the selection of new strains of viruses finally producing the various members of the pox viruses such as smallpox, cowpox, ectromelia in mice, horse pox, etc.

Paleoepidemiology is quite a mature science so far as the larger parasites are concerned, for speculation as to the origins and evolutions of these has proceeded in almost every discipline. The progress made has been very uneven, so that no good theory has been forthcoming to explain the origins of the tapeworms, while the steps by which the flukes evolved their complex cycles are still not too clear. Most workers would accept the concept that arthropod-borne infections originated in the arthropod and not the vertebrate host, but later in this book the alternate possibility in the case of *Plasmodium* is expressed as being the more likely. When, however, the bacteria and viruses are approached, it is soon seen that in this area paleoepidemiology is a sadly neglected science. Not only is there lack of comparative factual evidence, which to a large extent is inevitable, but also poverty of the theoretical studies. Concepts on the evolution of organismal groups, such as the acid fast bacilli, the *Salmonellae,* and the coccal forms, are very much underdeveloped; the concept of a species still held by many, perhaps the great majority, of microbiologists is many decades behind that of zoologists and botanists. There is no unanimity as to the nature of viruses, whether they are organisms in their own right or sometimes merely fractions of larger cells. Fortunately, the somewhat sterile discussions as to whether viruses are living or dead, which was stimulated by the discovery that they could be crystallized, seem to have abated.

A purpose of this book is to demonstrate that studies of infections in prehistory and the utilization of speculation in this and other epidemiologic research are possible, practical, and of value in tackling the field problems of today. The theoretical aspects include the various theories given later in the book; the practical uses of such thinking can be seen in the approach to infections such as cholera, the classification and nomenclature of microorganisms, and the studies on eradication. This chapter will be devoted to a brief catalogue of the materials and theories of general science lying waiting to be exploited by the student of paleoepidemiology.

In neoepidemiology, the "horizontal" epidemiology of the present day, the data available are usually of a type that can be measured. Time itself can be accurately broken down into days, hours, or minutes; the hosts and pathogens can not only be named and placed into recognized biological species, but can also be counted; various indicators of infection such as serologic tests can be employed and the titers estimated down to the last power. Statistical methods of great elegance and ingenuity have been devised to analyze this mass of scientific facts; the geography of the world has been estimated down to the last fifty feet, and the climatic variations are recorded continuously in innumerable places on the globe.

In paleoepidemiology, the vertical and horizontal epidemiology of the past, the position is greatly different, for the evidence that can be used is more qualitative than quantitative. One discusses the nature of things rather than their number. The time factor is usually obscure, the species of the host is known only by a few fossils or mummified remains or by philosophical reasoning; with rare exceptions, there are no pathogens to be identified physically, serology does not yet exist, population figures are unknown, temperatures and environment can be estimated only in a gross sort of fashion. Even the geography is uncertain so that, for example, there is still some question as to the age in which Australia was last joined to Asia, or whether Australia was ever linked to South America. In spite of this, there is still a surprising amount of data that can be used, so that the general picture of the spread of infection can be "blocked in" with some confidence, and doubtless as science progresses more and more details will be uncovered. The type of data that is available can be grouped into written and pictorial records, human relicts, paleobacteriology and serology, and the resources of modern biology in general.

Written records

The earliest seem to be those of the Chinese, going back 4,000 or 5,000 years (1). Unfortunately, very few have been translated into modern languages, and so are not accessible to students of the Western world. In addition, the forms in which diseases were described were not in the objective manner of Hippocrates, with an account of sign and symptoms, but were clothed in theoretical terms to such an extent that it is difficult at the present time to understand to what infection the author was referring. A recent work by Hoeppli is a good example of what is available (2). However, smallpox and tuberculosis were clearly described and variolation against smallpox was in use by A.D. 1000 (3).

Rabies was one of the first diseases to be recorded in writing. "Perhaps the earliest reference to it occurs in the Pre-Mosaic Eshnunna Code which predates the better known Code of Hammurabi of ancient Babylon in the 23rd century B.C. In this Code, the following excerpt is found: 'If a dog is mad and the authorities have brought the fact to the knowledge of its owner; if he does not keep it in, it bites a man and causes his death, then the owner shall pay two-thirds of a mina (40 shekels) of silver. If it bites a slave and causes his death he shall pay 15 shekels of silver' " (4).

From the tombs of Egypt have come many writings on papyrus that give accounts of medical practice thousands of years ago. Some are written in very clear and objective styles so that the conditions can often be recognized today. For example, the instructions for the surgical treatment of trichiasis permit a diagnosis of trachoma to be made.

The Ayurvedic system of medicine is still flourishing in India and Ceylon. The most widely used book is the ten volume text compiled by Susruta about 3,000 years ago. In Ceylon, Ayurvedic physicians drew my attention to descriptions of smallpox, infectious hepatitis, and malaria in the ancient texts they were using. They translated the Sanscrit and Pali into Singhalese and thence into English, giving adequate accounts of these diseases written about 3,000 years ago. The treatment recommended for infectious hepatitis was on dietary lines and much the same as that of today, while there was a passage that suggested that malaria was transmitted by small biting insects.

The Indians recognized smallpox long before Christ, and there is an ancient cult of smallpox worshipers in Central India, centered on a hill whose rocky outcrops from a distance resemble smallpox lesions. Relatives of sufferers of the disease even today do a kind of penance and crawl on hands and knees for considerable distances to the hill to appease the god.

Hippocrates describes many recognizable infections including pulmonary tuberculosis, malaria, erysipelas, and mumps, so that we know that these were present in Grecian days (5). In Roman times, Galen reported on plague (6), and in the days of Justinian there was a great epidemic of the infection that killed off a very substantial proportion of the population. Celsus not only gave a good picture of rabies, but even suggested that it was due to a virus, the term "virus" at that time meaning a "venom" (7).

From Roman times on, there are masses of writings that have been little studied, and which would provide the raw material of epidemiologic efforts. The Arab physicians, such as Razes, and the monks of the Middle Ages wrote much that was excellent for its time— Razes, for instance, gave the first account of measles, although he confused it somewhat with smallpox. However, the research worker in this field must not only be a physician but also familiar with the language and customs of the people he is studying. For example, the word "leprosy" has changed much in meaning since biblical times. Apparently the word in the original Jewish sense had a religious rather than medical meaning, while the term "measles" first meant leprosy. In any event, it is unlikely that the descriptions of diseases given in the Bible were all due to Hansen's disease, but may have been a mixed batch of skin lesions, including fungus infections and psoriasis. There is a school of thought that thinks that the leprosy in ancient times was really syphilis and that about 1490 the name was merely changed, so explaining the sudden appearance of "syphilis" and the simultaneous disappearance of leprosy in Europe about that time.

In Ceylon I made an error of this kind. In Kandy a palm leaf was seen on which was written in Pali an account of an epidemic of long ago. The monk who was translating the ancient writing into Singhalese stated that "a red-eyed demon visited the villages and many people died," and the accompanying Singhalese physician who acted as interpreter added that the disease in question was malaria, the introduction of which to Ceylon was partially blamed for the downfall of the early civilization. At the time, a mental reservation was made that conjunctivitis must have been a prominent feature of this ancient epidemic, though what eye infection could be associated with a killing disease of this kind I did not know. The matter was resolved a year later, when a collection of devil masks was seen. Each of the main diseases had its own devil mask, made in the likeness of the particular devil, and used to chase away that devil. That for malaria had red eyes. The "red-eyed demon" referred to the devil mask, and not the clinical condition.

Explorers sometimes gave reports of infectious diseases, so that we know that the Australian aborigines had trachoma because Dampier, the first Englishman on that continent, recorded that the natives sometimes had to throw their heads back to see out of their eyes, a condition that still exists there to this day. However, the passage is capable of other interpretations, and some believe that trachoma was recently introduced by traders (8, 9). Cortez wrote to the Spanish king to say that sometimes the people of the New World were "coloured"—i.e., had "pinta." Captain Cook remarked that the people of Hawaii were infected with yaws before the white man got there; indeed some of his sailors became infected (10). There are several reports of the Spanish introduction of smallpox to the New World, the most authoritative being the eye witness account by Diaz (11).

Pictorial Records

The oldest known pictorial records are the incredible paintings and drawings executed by men during the Ice Age in the caves of Spain and South France. They are as fresh today as when first done about 15,000 years ago. Unfortunately, for our purposes, they are limited largely to animals, although there is one in the Grotte de Lascaux which depicts a man being killed by a bull. Similar paintings, but of a more recent period, are now being discovered in Africa and Australia, and a search of these might reveal conditions of value in paleoepidemiology.

In more recent times, the Egyptians and other races have drawn many portraits from life and these enable diagnoses to be made in favorable circumstances. The best known is a probable case of poliomyelitis shown in Plate II, which is the first indication we have as to the placing in time and place of this infection. As time passed, the likenesses came to resemble the sitters with increasing accuracy, so that when Oliver Cromwell wanted an exact reproduction, "Warts and all," a record was made of a viral infection.

In South America, some groups of Indians or pre-Columbian days had the delightful custom of making their water pots in the form of human figures in various attitudes. More than 500 of these pots have been collected and some of them show infections quite clearly. One such pot depicts a person removing chiggers from the feet, another is of a hunchback possibly with Pott's disease, while several include representations of Leishmania infection (12).

Human Relicts

Most races of humans take special care of the dead body and often bury the remains in cemeteries. For obvious reasons there are difficulties in examining the more recent materials from this source, but cemeteries would be the major source of information for our purpose in the future. All over the world are lying samples of populations from different eras, and these will tell us not only a good deal of the infections which the people suffered from, but also will reveal the age distribution at the time of death.

The best data come from Egypt where people were mummified after death for the express purpose of preserving the body. In this process, the internal organs were removed and often placed in preserving fluid of a fixative nature in a pot at the side of the body. From such specimens it has been possible to diagnose pneumonias and smallpox by lesions in the respective tissues, and even to demonstrate bacteria in sections. Numerous cases of tuberculosis have been found, including one mummy of a priest of Ammon with a lesion in a vertebra and a psoas abscess. In the bladder of one person were clearly recognizable *Schistosoma haematobium* eggs, the earliest record of this to date (13).

In China and Japan are vast cemeteries that have arisen as a result of ancestor worship; all over Europe are great cemeteries that have been carefully preserved; and even in America are great sources of material, for the Indians there commonly grouped their dead together. In Canada, for instance, some tribes at frequent intervals used to congregate, bearing the bones of those dead since the previous meeting and with ceremony buried these in one common grave. Of course, the information gathered from such material is sharply limited to those infections causing pathology in bones, although as will be mentioned, there are possibilities of using more refined methods of diagnosis. Even with this limitation it has been possible to diagnose, for example, treponemal infections from bones from many parts of the world, including ancient ones from Iraq and the Polynesian Islands of the Pacific.

Occasional discoveries are made of bodies in unusual conditions of preservation, and these permit more precise examinations. For example, in Peru, a body 4,000 years old was found that had been mummified accidentally by climatic conditions; some of the hair was still attached to the skull and on this were the eggs of head lice, the earliest known record of this parasite (14). Also in this region was found a few years ago the frozen body of a boy who had been sacrificed to the mountain gods. His body had been placed in a stone chamber on top of a mountain where it had remained frozen ever since. It was removed to the plains in a refrigerated condition and on careful examination whipworm eggs were found in the intestine (15). In the Arctic, there must be many such bodies lying preserved in the frozen condition. Some years ago, in Alaska an imaginative, although unsuccessful, attempt was made to explore this by attempting to recover influenza virus. Large numbers of Eskimos had died of influenza during the great 1918 pandemic, and their bodies had sometimes been buried in common graves in the permafrost layer of soil. In the hope that the 1918 strain of influenza virus might still be recoverable, some of the bodies were dug up and tested, unfortunately without success. Such efforts are not unreasonable, as might seem at first sight, for it is a well-known fact that tissues and organisms are preserved for long periods under such conditions. Many frozen bodies of animals like mammoths have been preserved in the frozen soil of the Arctic, although the tale of the mammoth of northern Russia of 50 years ago that was taken to Moscow in the frozen state and served up at a special banquet (the mammoth steak was said to taste a little musty) is unfortunately without foundation (16). A few years ago, another small mammoth was found in Alaska and taken to New York in two refrigerators, where the plants it had been eating so long ago were still identifiable in its stomach.

Paleobacteriology and Serology

In the nineteenth century, Virchow pointed out that bacteria could be demonstrated in the bones of fossils of very great age, and this had been amply confirmed. Sometimes the fossils have pathologic lesions and the bacteria can be seen associated with these. The claim for the oldest known bacteria has been made for some micrococci in the rocks of Wyoming, dating back many hundreds of millions of years. Walcott was testing the theory that the rocks had been laid down partly as the result of the activity of bacteria and prepared thin sections of the rock and found these cocci in them (17). Since then, a search has been made for signs of life in the pre-Cambrian rocks from which fossils are absent and morphologically identifiable algae and primitive bacteria have been demonstrated. These rocks are about two billion years old (18).

A most intriguing discovery with regard to fossils is that not only are the morphologic outlines of creatures preserved in rocks, but also much of their chemical make-up. By means of chromatography, it is possible to examine the fossils of 300 million years ago and extract from them the amino acids that presumably were originally contained in their bodies (19). Amino acids appear to be stable over very long periods of time, provided that there is no excessive heat, and perhaps proteins may survive very much longer than had been thought possible. If this is so, then there is a likelihood of testing ancient human bones or older fossils for antibodies, and fossil bacteria for antigens. Something in this line has already been commenced with the blood grouping of mummies thousands of years old. Indeed, in a recent review of such blood grouping and the discussion that followed, it was pointed out that one of the difficulties was the substances from contaminating bacteria that could give nonspecific positives (20, 21). If blood group antigens can survive so long, then perhaps other antigens do the same. Incidentally, good blood group reactions can be obtained from bones, which encourages the idea that serologic studies can be carried out successfully on the most abundant relict material available. If antigens survive preserved in bacteria, then the typing of ancient organisms may be practical.

General Biology

There are great resources in general biology that can be utilized by the paleoepidemiologist, in the form of general principles as well as specific theories. In the succeeding chapters will be given several examples of the manner in which these can be applied to infectious diseases. Eight theories are studied in some detail, none of them original, but all being adapted from those existing in other disciplines in biology. These are listed as follows:

1. All parasites are descended from free-living organisms.
2. Man, in common with other members of the primate radia-

tion, has many parasites derived from those of the original ancestor of the radiation. These human parasites are therefore closely related to those of present-day apes, monkeys, and other primates.

3. Populations tend to acquire an increasing resistance of a genetically transmitted, non-specific character to their parasites.

4. For each infection and set of circumstances, there is a minimum threshold of host population; if the population falls below this threshold, the infection will die out. As a result, the acuteness of an infection is related to the size of the "herd"; small, isolated populations have chronic infections and large ones have more acute infections.

5. The "crowd infections" have arisen in the past few thousand years as a result of the population explosion resulting from the agricultural revolution.

6. Many crowd infections are derived from the infections of the animals in man's ecology.

7. Isolation of a population modifies its infectious diseases.

8. Some vector-borne infections, notably malaria, originated in the vertebrate.

REFERENCES

1. WONG, K. C. AND WU, L. T.: *A History of Chinese Medicine.* Tientsin Press, China, 1932
2. HOEPPLI, R.: *Parasites and Parasitic Infections in Early Medicine and Science.* Univ. of Malaya Press, Singapore, 1959.
3. ROLLESTON, J. D.: *History of the Acute Exanthemata.* Heineman, London, 1937.
4. SELLERS, T. F.: "Rabies" in *Principles of Internal Medicine,* 2nd ed., T. R. Harrison, ed., McGraw-Hill, New York, 1954.
5. *Genuine Works of Hippocrates,* trans. by Francis Adams. Wood, New York, 1849.
6. *Galen:* A translation by R. M. Green. Charles C Thomas, Springfield, Ill., 1951.
7. CELSUS, AULUS CORNELIUS: *De Medicina,* trans. by W. G. Spencer, Harvard Univ. Press, Cambridge, Mass., 1935–38.
8. CLELAND, J. B.: Disease among the Australian aborigine. J. Trop. Med. & Hyg., 1928, **31:** 53–59, 66–70, 141–45, 157–60, 173–77.
9. MANN, I.: Probable origins of trachoma in Australasia. Bull. W.H.O., 1957, **16:** 1165–87.
10. COOK, J. AND KING, J.: *A Voyage to the Pacific Ocean.* Stockdale, London, 1784.
11. DIAZ, BERNAL: *The Bernal Diaz Chronicles,* trans. by Albert Idell, Dolphin Books. Doubleday & Co., New York, 1956.
12. MOODIE, R. L.: *The Antiquity of Disease.* Univ. of Chicago Press, Chicago, 1923.
13. RUFFER, SIR MARC ARMAND: *Studies in Palaeopathology of Egypt.* Univ. of Chicago Press, Chicago, 1921.

14. EWING, H. E.: American lice of the genus *Pediculus*. Proc. U.S. Nat. Mus., 1926, **68:** 1–30.
15. PIZZI, T. AND SCHENONE, H.: Trichuris in an Inca. Trop. Med. & Hyg. News, 1955, **42.**
16. FARRAND, W. R.: Frozen mammoths and modern geology. Science, 1961, **133:** 729–35.
17. WALCOTT, C. D.: The discovery of Algonkian bacteria. Proc. Nat. Acad. Sci., 1915, **1:** 256.
18. BRIGGS, M. H.: Dating the origin of life on earth. Evolution, 1959, **13:** 416–18.
19. ABELSON, P. H.: Paleobiochemistry. Sci. Amer., 1956, **195:** 83–93.
20. SPRINGER, G. F. AND WILLIAMSON, P.: Blood group determinations of ancient tissues, Science, 1960, **131:** 1858.
21. SMITH, M.: Blood groups of ancient dead. Science, 1960, **131:** 699–702.

CHAPTER 4

The Evolution of
Infectious Diseases

Theory 1. All parasites are descended from free-living organisms.

THIS IS NO NEW theory. Many scientists have mentioned it, but most did so merely in passing and without any further discussion than just stating it (1, 2). And indeed there is really very little to be said about it in a general way.

If there is any truth in the theories of the origin of life that have already been discussed, then all biological systems must have been small and discrete in the beginning, while any form of symbiosis, from commensalism to extreme pathogenicity, would have been a secondary development. The only other possibility, that parasites have never lived independent lives but split off from their hosts, cannot be seriously considered: imagine, if you can, how that could have happened in the case of helminths, protozoa, or bacteria.

Viruses may perhaps be an exception to this rule, but many may not be parasites at all, only essential parts of the systems in which they are found. They can carry genetic material and inheritable characteristics from one "host" to another and may possibly be a kind of mobile gene, playing a vital part in the survival of their cells. This would be quite a logical development if life actually began in free-living biological systems the size of viruses, with more complex cells developing from some of them later. Such a theory would not invalidate the concept that viruses might arise from bacteria parasitic on cells, bacteria that have lost their capacity for independent life, for this could be the origin of some viruses like the psittacosis group and the rickettsiae.

For many kinds of parasites it is possible to arrange examples of related organisms in arrays, beginning at one end with that which is most highly dependent on its host, then proceeding down the line with those less dependent, and finishing up with a free-living organism. So for instance, one can start with the malaria parasite, a highly dependent parasite with a complex life cycle, including phases in the liver and red blood cells and transmission by an insect vector. The next step illustrating less complexity is shown by *Hepatocytes* in which the major reproduction of the parasites takes place in the liver, and the red cells are utilized mainly as vehicles for helping the parasites reach the vector. Next comes a protozoa that misses the liver altogether, in the form of *Schellackia,* a reptilian infection in which the reproduction takes place entirely in the intestine, the infective forms being carried directly to the skin by the blood where they are picked up by the mite vector. Return to the intestine occurs when the reptile swallows the mite. The vector-less stage is best demonstrated by *Eimeria,* a parasite of the intestine with a developmental cycle so like that of *Plasmodium* that by analogy it first suggested the life cycle of *Plasmodium* to the early pioneers investigating that infection. One can imagine easily how an intracellular parasite arose from a free-living form, for it is normal for the phagocytic cells of the host to engulf invaders, and some of these that find themselves inside of the phagocyte might be preadapted to survive there. That such a proceeding is not too uncommon is well demonstrated by the numerous bacilli that can survive in this fashion, including the tubercule bacillus, the meningococcus, and the gonococcus. Evolution of the complex sexual cycle of *Eimeria* is more difficult to illustrate by example, but there is nothing difficult in understanding it in a general way. That free-living protozoa have a form of sex life has been well demonstrated, being worked out in most detail for *Paramecium* (3). The procedure by which a free-living form comes in contact with the cells of the host's tissue has been discussed earlier in the section on symbiosis. In this fashion the process of development can be illustrated step by step by a series of analogies, beginning with the free-living form of protozoa and finishing up with the *Plasmodium* with its highly complex cycle in which at one time or another it parasitizes cells of the liver, blood, and mosquito. The question as to whether this occurred first in the vertebrate or the insect vector is argued in a later chapter.

Similarly, it is possible to array for many other parasites analogies for the intermediate steps in the evolutionary process. For the bacteria, as for many parasites, the change involves apparently the loss of various functions as the degree of parasitism deepens and some of these are listed in Chapter 5 on "The Species Concept in Microbiology." As described by Bissett, bacteria of the genus *Neissera* can be arrayed from the free-living Gram positive *Sarcinae* equipped with flagellum and spore down to the Gram negative obligate anaerobic and very small parasite *Veillonellay* (4).

Similarly, with the nematodes, an array can be set up, beginning with the free-living ones that are so common in the soil and water, then those that live in the intestine of animals but which have at least a partial period of free-living existence, to those which have invaded the tissues of their hosts, and finally to the nematodes that have evolved complex life cycles involving various arthropod vectors or invertebrate intermediate hosts.

The histories of the flukes and tapeworms are much more obscure (5), but there can be little doubt that in the beginning their ancestors were free-living animals. Sometimes clues to the nature of such ancestors are available; for example, the Linguatulidae, which are parasites of snakes with a superficial resemblance to tapeworms, and in the larval stages have four legs suggesting that an arthropod such as a mite might have been the original ancestor.

Theory 2. Many human parasites are modifications of those of the remote ancestral primate from which man, apes, monkeys, and other primates are descended.

There is nothing new in this theory which is well known to zoologists in general and parasitologists and taxonomists in particular. Von Thering is usually credited with first proposing the general principle about fifty years ago as applied to all animals, and Cameron has been a leading exponent of the concept in the last two decades (6). Recently in 1957, a symposium on the subject and labeled "Host Specificity among Parasites of Vertebrates" was held in Basel, Switzerland (7).

Theoretically, when populations of a species become isolated from each other, either geographically, ecologically, or genetically, and thus commence the evolutionary steps that lead to speciation (8), the parasites to which they are hosts will continue to exist in the new species and genera that develop. Since most of the variations that appear in the hosts will be structural rather than physiological, the parasites will remain in a fairly stable environment and thus will change less than their hosts do. The result will be that, although the related hosts may have markedly different appearances, yet these inherited parasites will continue much as before. Related hosts will therefore have the same or closely related parasites. When all or most of the species descended from one common stock are host to a

parasite that is not found outside that particular radiation, except
in a distantly related form, then it seems logical that these parasites
are derived from one that was on the ancestral host at the beginning
of the radiation.

Since man belongs to the adaptive radiation of the primates, we
could expect that he would have parasites in common with other
members of the order (Figure 4), and a good case can be made out
for some organisms having evolved in this way—the louse *Pediculus,*
of which several species have been reported from many primates

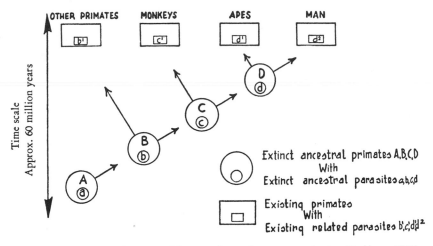

Figure 4. Parallel phylogenies of hosts and parasites among primates (Cockburn 1959)

but from no other animal (9, 10, 11, 12), *Enterobius,* the pin- or
threadworm, which has so far been found only in primates (13, 14),
and the intestinal protozoa, where there is usually no morphological
difference between those of man and those of monkey. Of the 14
protozoa commonly found in man, 13 are also found in apes and
monkeys (Table 4) (14–22). Primate malarial parasites of the genus
Plasmodium may also have arisen in the same way, for though there
are many species of the parasite infecting many vertebrate hosts, yet
the primate species form a separate group (23), within which there
is a definite correlation between relationships in the phylogenetic
tree of the hosts and the parasites. That is, the ape parasites are almost indistinguishable morphologically from human ones (24, 25),
those of the monkey are not quite so similar, and those of other
primates are even more dissimilar.

Among the viruses, the monkeys and apes have two that are closely related to man and which so far have been found in no other creatures. Herpes virus is an infection of man, having the peculiar characteristic of lying dormant after the initial infection, but being able to be reactivate and produce pathogenic effects when the host is exposed to conditions such as raised temperature or excessive sunlight. The equivalent monkey virus is the Sabin B virus which also lies dormant. In monkeys it causes only mild lesions such as ulcers

TABLE 4. INTESTINAL PROTOZOA OF PRIMATES

Protozoa of man	Man % infected (1)	Wild *M. philippenensis,* % infected (2)	Captive monkeys in China % infected (3)	Captive monkeys in London (4)	Other records from monkeys —captive (5)
E. histolytica	10	23	90	X	Dobell 1931
E. coli	50	50	60	X	Dobell 1919
					Dobell & Laidlaw 1926
E. gingivalis	50	84	—	—	Kofoid 1929
Endolimax nana	25	50	90	X	Craig & Faust 1945
Dientamoeba fragilis	?	5	—	X	
Trichomonas hominis	5–20	84	10	X	Dobell 1934
T. buccalis	10–30	84	—	—	
T. vaginalis	10–50 (women)	5	—	—	Dobell 1926
Giardia lamblia	10	14	10	X	Hegner 1924 Wenyon 1926
Chilomastrix mesnili	10	39	35	X	Hegner 1924
Balantidium coli	?	17	—	X	Brooks 1902 Brumpt 1909 Faust 1945
Iodamoeba williamsi	10	0	65	—	

(1) Hegner R. 1929 (17)
(2) Hegner R. & Chu H. J. 1930 (18)
(3) Kessel J. F. 1927 (21)

(4) Proc. Zool. Soc. London 1940–6
(5) Craig & Faust 1945

in the mouth (26), but should the infection be passed to man by the bite of a monkey the effects are much more serious. All the human cases so far reported have been fatal.

Infectious hepatitis and its presence in apes has not yet been fully studied, but the story is a strange one. The virus of this disease defied isolation until recent years, and even now a satisfactory means of growing it is not available. In spite of repeated inoculations of presumably infected materials from patients with the disease, the infection has not been transmitted to any laboratory animal. Within the past year, however, reports have appeared in which zoo and laboratory personnel have developed infectious hepatitis when handling chimpanzees, and once this was published it was quickly realized that this was indeed a serious hazard to such people. There seems little doubt that the chimpanzees at least can carry the infection, and judging from the widespread distribution of the reports, they probably did not get it from man but probably had it in the wild state. Whether the virus is identical to that of man or is somewhat different is not yet known (27).

Though we have confined our theory to the primate radiation, which is of comparatively recent origin, it also may apply to earlier radiations, such as that of the mammals or of the vertebrates. Salivary gland viruses could be a possible example of organisms derived from an ancestral parasite of the common mammalian ancestor, for they have been found in almost all animals tested so far—man, ape, monkey, rat, mouse, hamster, guinea pig, mole—and each virus is strictly specific for its own host with none being transmissible to unusual hosts. In spite of this, the similarities are great—type of inclusion body, cell reaction, etc.—which would easily indicate their common ancestry. However, little in the way of antigenic relationship has yet been found, except that, significantly, chimpanzee serum has complement-fixing antibodies against the human virus and the chimpanzee virus will grow in human cell tissue culture (28).

Plasmodium, which we have already discussed, could have derived from an organism that infected a common vertebrate ancestor, since it is found in almost all land animals and the various parasite species are not generally transmissible to vertebrates outside their normal host range (29). Even further back we may have the ancestor of both land and sea vertebrates parasitized by the ancestor of acid-fast organisms of the genus *Mycobacterium,* since it is found in both with a radiation parallel to that of its hosts. The human representative would be *Mycobacterium leprae,* for it is theorized later that *Mycobacterium tuberculosis* has been acquired from cattle at a more recent time.

Theory 3. Populations tend to become genetically resistant to their pathogens.

Infection with a pathogen reduces the survival capacity of the host, and all other factors being equal, the host with the most resistance is the one most likely to survive. If this resistance is inherited, then natural selection can be expected to produce a population more and more resistant to the prevalent pathogens, and in time a benign host-pathogen relationship will be established.*

The existence of genetically controlled non-specific resistance has been debated for more than 30 years, chiefly by two teams of workers, one in the United States led by Webster (30, 31) and another in England under Topley and Greenwood (32, 33). In 1923, Webster showed that mice varied in their resistance to infection with *Salmonella* species and that selective breeding would produce, from a strain of mice 40 per cent susceptible to infection, strains that were either 10 per cent or 90 per cent susceptible. In 1936, Greenwood and his colleagues (33) summarized their results as follows:

> The available experimental data appear to have established quite clearly the existence of significant differences in resistance between strains within the same species, e.g., between different strains of mice or rats. They strongly support the view that genetic differences in resistances exist within a strain, and that these differences can be segregated by selective breeding in such a way as to allow the production of derived strains of relatively high or relatively low resistance. . . . Taking the most favorable records, however, there is no instance in which animals of the selected strain were uniformly resistant to bacterial infection, even when the test of resistance was the injection of the bacteria concerned in a dose that failed to kill 100 per cent of the unselected controls.

This deficiency was made up by Sabin (34) in 1952, when he found a strain of mice that was 100 per cent resistant to a dosage of yellow fever virus that was 100 per cent lethal to standard test animals. By

---

* The earliest record I can find expressing this idea is contained in an article by W. C. Wells, who in 1813 read a paper before the Royal Society "An Account of a White female, part of whose skin resembles that of a Negro." In this paper Wells distinctly recognizes the principle of natural selection, and Darwin gives him full recognition to the prior claim of the discovery. After remarking that Negroes and mulattoes enjoy an immunity from certain tropical diseases, he observes, firstly, that all animals tend to vary in some degree, and secondly, that agriculturists improve their domesticated animals by selection; and then, he adds that what is done in this latter case by art seems to be done with equal efficacy, though more slowly, by nature, in the formation of varieties of mankind, fitted for the country which they inhabit. Of the accidental varieties of man which would occur among the first few and scattered inhabitants of the middle regions of Africa, some one would be better fitted than the others to bear the diseases of the country. This race would consequently multipy, while the others would decrease; not only from their inability to sustain the attacks of disease, but from their incapacity of contending with their more vigorous neighbors. (Charles Darwin. *The Origin of Species*. 6th ed. John Murray, London, 1906.)

cross-mating on Mendelian lines, he was able to show that this resistance was inherited according to Mendel's laws.

A most dramatic example of inherited non-specific resistance and natural selection in action has been provided in the past decade by the attempt to eliminate rabbits in Australia and Europe by loosing myxomatosis virus among them. This virus is derived from one that causes an enzootic non-fatal disease among rabbits of the American genus *Sylvilagus*. It is transmitted by mosquitoes in Australia and by rabbit fleas in Europe. Among Australian and European rabbits (which are of the same stock), first exposure to infection kills off 99 per cent of the herd in 10 to 12 days, but later exposure of descendants of the survivors results in a mortality of only 90 per cent, with the rabbits lingering 20 or 30 days before dying. This is due partly to the appearance of attenuated strains of virus, but also to the natural selection of genetically resistant animals. It seems only a matter of time before the disease becomes comparatively non-fatal in Australia and Europe as it already is in America (35).

This genetically inherited resistance to infection must be one of the fundamental factors in host-parasite relations. Examples can be seen on all sides, although it is not easy to delimit precisely the extent of the influence of this factor in any specific instances. In cattle, there is great variation in the resistance by strains to the infections found in their areas. It is notorious that the European cattle introduced to a tsetse fly infected country in Africa have very poor chances of surviving, while the native cattle are very little affected by the trypanosomes. There is obviously a number of factors involved in this, but undoubtedly the native cattle are born resistant and would be so whether previously exposed or not, while the European ones rapidly succumb on first exposure. It is the same story with rinderpest vaccine. This is excellent for some breeds but will cause considerable mortality in others, such as the European breeds and especially the highly susceptible Japanese black cattle which have little natural exposure to the natural infection. On the other hand, if vaccines are made suitable for these more susceptible breeds—it can be made using either goats, rabbits, or chick embryos—the resultant strains give a poor take on zebu cattle and even more so for buffalo (36).

Resistance to malaria due to the possession of an abnormal hemoglobin in the human being can be given as an example of non-specific genetically inherited resistance. The abnormal hemoglobin, which is responsible for a familial disease called sicklemia, is mildly disadvantageous to its possessors who, through natural selection, tend to be eliminated from non-malarious areas. However, because the malaria parasite seems to have difficulty in metabolizing the abnormal hemoglobin, in hyperendemic regions the mild handicap of sicklemia is more than counterbalanced by resistance to the parasite. This is said to be the reason why Negroes and others surviving in malarious areas have so high a carrier rate of the abnormal hemoglobin and the associated sicklemia (37).*

The development of genetic resistance in human beings may be as fast comparatively as that of rabbits to myxomatosis, clearly illustrated by the reaction to tuberculosis of the Indians in Saskatchewan (38, 39). When the buffalo disappeared in 1879, Indians were settled on reservations by the Canadian government and treaty money was paid, which meant that a census was kept. Before that date the Indians had been completely nomadic, having little contact with traders and, as far as is known, little or no tuberculosis. To quote Ferguson, the authority on the subject, it was "uncommon and unimportant as a cause of death."

After 1879 the picture changed. A most disastrous epidemic appeared among the tribes settled on the reservations, and within a few years the general death rate among them was varying from 90 to 140 deaths per 1,000, two thirds of them due to tuberculosis. The first accurate figures are for 1882 when the epidemic was already under way, the death rate being about 20/1000, rising rapidly to 90/1000 in 1896, and then gradually subsiding to about 8/1000 in the 1930's, which was about 20 times the rate for the surrounding white population. At present, the mortality is approaching that of the surrounding white population.

This severe and prolonged epidemic can be attributed to many causes: inadequate diet after the disappearance of the buffalo, poor housing, overcrowding, and general spiritual demoralization. Yet many Europeans, exposed to conditions as bad as those of the In-

---

* Resistance to many infections is obviously related to Gamma Globulin concentration. The total lack of Gamma Globulin is clearly dependent on genetic factors, while differences in levels may be due to racial, nutritional, or exposure to infections in general. Children exposed to repeated infection with malaria parasites have marked increases in serum Gamma Globulin concentrations. Healthy adult Gambians turn over Gamma Globulin at a daily rate that is eight times that of Europeans. It has long been known that "crowding out" of antibody formation may take place if an antigen is injected into an animal when active production of another antibody is occurring. Possibly, therefore, a population that is exposed to one heavy infection may respond poorly to a later exposure to some other pathogen. (McGregor, I. A. and Barr, M.: Antibody response to tetanus toxoid inoculation in malarious and non-malarious children. Trans. Roy. Soc. Trop. Med. Hyg. 1962, 56: 364–66.)

dians, do not have mortality figures of this magnitude, suggesting that they have developed higher resistance during their long exposure to infection. In working out family trees for the Indian reservations, Ferguson found that though all families were infected during the epidemic, some survived with not too high a mortality, while others were wiped out completely. The present stock is, of course, descended from the survivors, and the part played by natural selection in so few generations must have been a large one.

In man, there are substantial variations in the reactions to yellow-fever virus. In its endemic home in Africa, the native populations are highly resistant and the infection is to a large extent a silent one. Surveys, using the mouse-protection test for the detection of antibodies, indicate that up to 50 per cent or more of a population have antibodies in a certain area, yet there may have been little or no disease (40).

The difficulty of finding and diagnosing yellow fever in the native African is well illustrated by the experience of the Entebbe group in Bwamba County. Here again the protection test indicated that the disease had been present within recent years, but the most careful search by experienced workers failed to reveal a single case during a four-year study. It was only after the protection test demonstrated the existence of the disease, in a restricted area within recent months, that cases were found. The explanation for this lies, in part at least, in the fact that a high percentage of yellow-fever cases in Africans are so mild that they cannot be diagnosed clinically (40).

Severe and fatal cases of yellow fever, exhibiting the classic symptoms of the disease, do occur in Africa, but apparently they are rare.

It is quite a different story for the European or American. Contact with the virus does not produce the mild disease of the Africa of the endemic area, but a very serious and highly lethal disorder. History is full of accounts of white groups arriving in Africa and high percentages of them succumbing to the disease. It was the same story when the virus was introduced to susceptible populations in America. It is estimated that the epidemic that visited the Mississippi Valley in 1878 caused 13,000 deaths, while during that of 1905 in New Orleans and other ports of the South, there were 1,000 deaths in 5,000 cases, a mortality rate of 20 per cent (40).

The same picture, only in reverse, is seen in measles. Here it is the European who is highly resistant, and the African and those populations on remote islands who are highly susceptible. Measles in the temperate climates, which seems to have been its original endemic home, is a comparatively mild disease, and there are many inapparent infections. Although most Americans are infected sooner or later in life, usually by the end of the sixth or seventh year, yet the total number of deaths from the disease in the U.S. is only about 500 per year. In contrast, when the virus is introduced to communities that have not been previously exposed, the death rate is very high; such was the experience of the Indians of Central America and Peru in the early days of the Spaniards (41), or the peoples of Samoa and Hawaii in the nineteenth century (55). In West Africa today, measles is becoming one of the major causes of death.

It is usually said that this high death rate in Africa, Hawaii, and Samoa was the result of lack of medical care and treatment. There is a certain amount of justification for this statement, but my experience is that it is only a minor part of the story. In 1935, I was in practice in Bedlington, a coal-mining town in the north of England, during a particularly heavy epidemic of measles, and on my morning rounds on foot, would call at practically every house down the long rows so typical of that part of the country. In one morning I would see fifty or more cases, for in almost every house there was one or more children with measles. Any treatment I could give was almost totally without effect, for these were the days before antibiotics, yet only one child died. There were lots of cases of pneumonia, running ears, and other such complications, but these were not fatal. The only time I saw high fatality rates in England were in London in 1937–38, while on the staff of the North Eastern Fever Hospital. One week my ward had several children with the mulberry form of the disease and there were a number of deaths. The following year, while working in public health in Barking, I saw an epidemic of measles with some pneumonia, which coincided with one of whooping cough, and there were a few deaths from the mixed infections. In West Africa in 1942–44, during my tour of duty there as hygiene specialist in the British Army, it was a different story. There were several outbreaks of the disease; the care and treatment the patients received did not differ in any essentials from that in northern England in the pre-antibiotic days, but the illnesses were much more severe and the deaths far more numerous. Many adults had the disease. English and African children are not strictly comparable, for there are marked differences in diet and, in addition, the African children carried a host of various parasites, but the difference in the severities of the measles was of a kind not explicable by such factors. It was simply a fact of variation in reaction to the virus.

An instance of apparent natural resistance to infection with schistosomes impressed me in West Africa. In that area, the Africans often, with very little discomfort, survived degrees of infection that would have overwhelmed Europeans. In 1943 I accompanied the late G. M. Findlay on a visit to some villages near the mouth of Volta River to collect specimens of *Schistosoma* eggs for experimental work on monkeys. The people of villages were well known to be heavily infected with the parasites, and a decade or so later were the subject of an intensive study (42). On arrival, we found a number of very shallow fresh water lakes with several villages on their banks. The men living there were fishermen who waded into the water to cast their nets, while the women collected water and washed their clothes in the lakes. All members of the communities, from the smallest child to the oldest adult, defecated or washed themselves in the lakes. Since the shallow waters at the edges were full of snails, it seemed a most likely place to find cases of schistosomiasis. Imagine, therefore, our surprise when at first we found none. The villagers looked at us with astonishment when asked if they suffered from symptoms of the disease and if they passed blood in their urine. They had heard of something similar to that which we described, but said they had seen nothing like it. For an hour the questioning went on with results that were completely negative. They simply insisted that they were not ill with this disease and never had been.

At this stage we asked if they would at least let us have samples of urine to examine, and a number of small boys obliged. The urine was heavily bloodstained and the color of port wine, so we asked the chief why he didn't tell us about the blood. He replied that there was no blood in the urine; urine was always this color in children, and there was nothing unusual in the specimens just passed! In fact, further examination showed that all the children were very heavily infected with the parasites, but none admitted to any symptoms in spite of the heavy blood loss and the excretion of eggs.

In contrast to this, there was an incident in which some British soldiers came into contact with cercariae and then the story was greatly different. It was during the time that the 81st and 82nd West African divisions were being trained for the fighting in Burma. The Africans had to be taught how to swim across rivers, but the difficulty was in finding a place to practice swimming that was free of crocodiles, sharks, and schistosomes. Finally, a lagoon on the coast was chosen because of its salt water, and training begun. What was not realized at the time was that a small stream entering at the far end did not merely mix with the salt water but swept along the shore as a band of fresh water in which fresh-water snails could live. The soldiers entering the lagoon for swimming practice went through this narrow, snail infested band of fresh water before entering the salt water. Sometime afterward, a number of troops developed signs of infection of a most virulent kind, including skin troubles due to the eggs becoming lodged in the skin capillaries. The reactions of the British troops were much more serious than those described above of the small children in the villages. This cannot be attributed entirely to any acquired immunity. The African resistance must have been due, partially at least, to natural selection of a marked kind, operating over many generations under conditions of continuous superinfection

Theory 4. The acuteness of an infection is related to the size of the "herd."

All other factors being equal, and providing that there is time enough for natural selection to operate, a large, isolated herd will tend to have many quick-spreading infections of short duration, and a small, isolated herd will have only chronic infections with low infectivity. If both acute and chronic types of the same infection were present in a large population at the same time, the acute one, because of its faster spread, would involve more people and leave only a minority group for the chronic variety. In a small population, the reverse would apply: the acute type would sweep through most of the susceptible persons and die out, but the chronic infection could linger on until more susceptible persons had appeared.*

In a very small population with few susceptible persons, the survival of a pathogen depends on its ability to exist until new hosts appear. Natural selection will therefore favor those that can live

---

* Many physicians have expressed this idea in one form or another. For example, Dr. W. H. Hamer in 1906 commented as follows with regard to the endemicity of influenza: "It is important to observe that the capacity for smouldering depends upon the existence of a large population densely aggregated. It may be roughly stated that in London, with its 5,000,000 people, some million cases occur up to the time of maximum prevalence; there are after 13 weeks some 5,000 cases a week; and a few cases still occur weekly even after six months. On this basis we see that in a population of say 5,000 persons, the outbreak would have practically terminated after 13 weeks, and be altogether extinct before the end of half a year. In these considerations we may find explanation of the behaviour of influenza in Martinique, Réunion, or the Fiji Islands." (Dr. W. H. Hamer. "Epidemic Diseases in England." *The Lancet,* 1906, p. 735).

in a kind of commensal relationship with their hosts and those that can continue to live away from their hosts. This would mean the following: no infections like measles, which spread rapidly and immunize a majority of the population in one epidemic, but many like typhoid, amoebic dysentery, pinta, trachoma, or leprosy, in which the host will remain infective for long periods of time, and others like malaria, filariasis, and schistosomiasis, where the infection not only persists in the host for a long time but also has an outside host to serve as an additional reservoir.

The effect of the introduction of an acute infection into a small, isolated community was first studied in 1846 by Panum, who collected much valuable data about disease in a small "herd" on the Faroe Islands off the northern coast of Scotland. He was studying an epidemic of measles, but included many other data, and they are appropriate for our purpose because the peoples of these islands formed a closed community, having only occasional contact with the outside world, and living under conditions very similar to those of the early hunting and fishing era. In 1846, when the population was 7,782, measles appeared suddenly and attacked nearly everyone. A previous epidemic in 1781 had also infected almost the whole population, but the disease had disappeared completely afterward, presumably owing to a lack of susceptible persons (43).

This time measles was brought to the islands by a carpenter who had been exposed to the disease just before leaving Copenhagen. He became sick in April, soon after his arrival at the islands, and by October the disease had spread everywhere, severely affecting people of all ages. The 92 persons who had been in the 1781 epidemic escaped infection in 1846. Some villages escaped by rigid quarantine and isolation, but 95.6 per cent of the rest of the population, about 6,000 persons of a possible 6,682, contracted measles. The infection then disappeared from the islands, again presumably owing to lack of susceptible persons (Table 5).

Panum also commented on the absence of other infectious diseases in the Faroes, except when brought in by outside visitors, and it is now well recognized that small, isolated groups like the coal miners on Spitsbergen or Arctic and Antarctic explorers are free from infections like the common cold and influenza just so long as they have no personal contact with the outside world, but are likely to succumb as soon as the first ship arrives. Even pathogens that can live in their hosts like commensals for months find it difficult to survive if the population is too small. Bodian said that poliomyelitis dies out in small communities after a certain time, even though carriers can excrete the virus for many months (44).

We still do not know what size population is needed in various types of civilization to support the different pathogens. Obviously a much larger herd is needed by acute infections that produce solid immunities and do not have carriers (a type of infection usually referred to here as "acute crowd infections") than is required by a disease like typhoid fever, where one person may excrete the organism for many decades. It is therefore suggested that in each infection and set of circumstances there is a minimum population that is necessary for its continued existence; if the herd falls below this threshold

TABLE 5. FAROE ISLANDS MEASLES EPIDEMIC, 1846

Age groups	Population	Number attacked	Deaths	Case fatality per cent
Under 1 year	198	154	44	28.6
1–9	1,440	1,117	3	0.3
10–19	1,525	1,183	2	0.2
20–29	1,470	1,140	4	0.3
30–39	842	653	10	1.5
40–49	791	613	19	3.1
50–59	728	565	27	4.8
60–69	480	372	27	7.3
70–79	272	211	19	9.0
80 and over	118	92	15	16.3
Total	7,864	6,100	170	2.8

level, the pathogen will die out. The larger the herd, the more acute and transient the infections it can support.

The manner in which a chronic infection can survive in a small community was well illustrated by an experience of mine in Massachusetts in 1955. At that time I was health officer for Berkshire County, a heavily wooded, mountainous area, composed of a large number of small townships. Some of these are quite remote and one township is so small that it has a permanent population of only 50 people, although the numbers swell in the summer to a hundred times this figure. In one of these townships a certain family had the reputation of being a "typhoid" family, for over the past 30 years, which was as far as the available records and peoples' memories could go, there had been a continual sequence of cases of that disease. The typhoid had appeared in the family as single cases at intervals of some years, and in the early 1940's there had been a small epidemic in the town that was traced back to the milk supplies from a farm belonging to this family.

In 1955 the old grandmother, aged 82, was admitted to the hospital for diabetes, and by chance a specimen of feces was examined. She was found to be a typhoid carrier and must have been one ever since the age of 18, when she contracted the infection from her father. On examining the records more closely, it became obvious that, in spite of the intensive studies made on the family, she had always somehow escaped scrutiny. For 66 years she had kept the infection alive in her small family group, spreading it to her husband, her sisters, children, grandchildren, and the people her children married, and at least once to the townspeople who drank the milk from her farm.

There is little in the way of precise and well-documented data on the infections of small groups of people living isolated existences under conditions of a hunting economy. The main difficulty now is finding such groups that have not already been infected as the result of contact with larger civilizations. About three decades ago, what was known about the infections of the Australian aborigines was written up by Cleland (45) and Basedow (46), and more recently Mann (47) has published work on the eye infections of these people. As would be expected, most of the infections reported are of a chronic nature, such as trachoma, malaria, irkinja, which is one of the treponematoses, and roundworms. However, obvious spread has taken place from the more recent colonists and traders, so that, for instance, an outbreak of smallpox was reported within a year of the first British settlement. It was said to have crossed the continent from the north and possibly was started by Malay fishermen. Even trachoma may have been introduced by the white traders, as maintained by Mann (48), although others think that Dampier, the first British explorer to reach Australia, was indeed describing the disease when he said that the natives had to throw their heads back to see straight ahead. Tuberculosis is apparently found predominantly only among those natives living in close association with the white man.

In Africa, Jelliffe and his colleagues have studied the infection of the Hadza (49). This is a hunting people of northern Tanganyika, about 800 in number and living an isolated life in the tsetse area of the savannah country. Their economy is entirely that of hunting and food gathering and they have very little contact with other peoples, who normally avoid living in this region because of the sleepy sickness. They are a click-speaking race, possibly allied to the Kung Bushmen of South West Africa and the cave painters of East Africa. They are very mobile especially in wet weather. They eat almost anything they can get including baboon, vulture, and hyena, but not tortoises. The food is usually barbecued.

An examination of 62 children showed them to be well nourished and with good teeth. Malaria parasites were present in 27 per cent. In the stools, four children had Taenia, which probably came from the wart hogs that they ate, and three had Giardia infection. Thirty per cent had conjunctivitis and many had ringworm. There were no roundworm or hookworm, presumably because the constant moving prevented transmission. In other words, their only infection found was that of a very chronic nature that could survive in a small population that was always on the move. Other infections such as measles, rubella, and chickenpox would come to them only as introduced infections, from populations large enough to support them on a permanent basis.

Theory 5. The acute crowd infections did not exist before the urbanization of society a few thousand years ago.

A number of writers, including Bates (50) and Bedson *et al.* (51), have expressed this theory in one form or another. Such infections are caused by pathogens that are very largely specific to human beings, have no other animal reservoir, are unable to survive for long periods away from their host, do not form commensal-like states with their host in the form of chronic disease or prolonged carrier phases, and exist solely by rapid transfer from one susceptible person to another. This definition covers measles, mumps, smallpox, chickenpox, rubella, the common cold, cholera, and possibly influenza. It is not strictly applicable to tuberculosis, but there is good reason to suppose that this is also a crowd disease, which has evolved in the same way and at the same time. Tuberculosis in a primitive society is an acute disease, as will be discussed later.

It would seem most unlikely that infections such as measles could have existed for any length of time in the small human communities of the hunting era, which are thought to have included not more than 600 persons at the most, for even though a pathogen of that type could have evolved, it would soon have exhausted the supply of susceptible persons and would then have become extinct. During the next era, however, when great cities and civilizations appeared and flourished, the population would pass the threshold level needed for the support of acute crowd infections. Unfortunately, our oldest records of this type of infection go back only two or three thousand years, so that there is no direct evidence for this belief and we must rely on indirect evidence.

The urbanization of man proceeded on a large scale only in certain areas of India, China, and the Middle East; until quite recently, Europe, Africa, America, and Australia were relatively underpopulated—England at the time of the Norman Conquest had only about one million inhabitants (52), and America at the time of Columbus only about eight million (53, 54), scattered almost from one pole to the other. In contrast to this, by 4000 B.C. some cities in Iraq housed 200,000 persons, so that acute crowd infections could be expected to have originated in those areas, spreading outward only after the development of modern communication.

Two kinds of evidence can be provided to support the thesis that the acute community infections originated in the crowded urban areas of the world and did not exist in the other parts until introduced there from outside. First, there is documentary and pathological evidence of the existence of infections like smallpox and tuberculosis in urban areas dating back long before Christ. Secondly, the conclusion that such diseases did not exist in the non-urban communities until introduced can be reached by showing that such communities were highly susceptible to them when contact with the rest of the world was first made. A community experiencing a new infection for the first time reacts differently from one that has suffered from it for a long time. All age groups will be affected, not only the children, and the death rate will be high, since natural selection will not have had time to build up the non-specific resistance to the pathogen. If this can be shown to happen consistently with the non-urban populations of the world, there is a good case for maintaining that these infections did not originate there.

First, there are plenty of descriptive writings from ancient times to show that infections like measles, smallpox, mumps, and tuberculosis existed in the Mediterranean regions and India and China long before the era of transoceanic travel commenced.

Smallpox is the earliest of the acute exanthemata to be accurately described. According to Rolleston (57), China is the home of smallpox and, although claims for its very early presence there are said to be discredited, it was undoubtedly in existence by A.D. 49 when the Huns invaded the country. In the reign of Chien Wu, about two hundred years later, we find in the "Handbook of Prescriptions for Emergencies" by the alchemist Ko Hung who lived in the Chin Dynasty (265–313 A.D.) the following description: "Recently there have been persons suffering from epidemic sores which have attacked the head, face and trunk. In a short time the sores spread over the body. They have the appearance of hot boils containing some dry matter. While some of the sores dry up a fresh crop appears. If it is not treated early the patient usually dies. Those that recover are disfigured by purplish scars which do not fade until after a year." (57).

Hirsch and other authorities view India as the original home of smallpox (55). Traditions concerning this disease have long existed among the Brahmins, and there has been temple worship of a deity whose protection was invoked on the outbreak of an epidemic. It has also been suggested that smallpox was the cause of an epidemic described by Quintus Curtius as occurring in the fourth century B.C. among the army of Alexander at the mouth of the Indus. ("Quippe scabies corporis invasit et contagium morbi etiam in alios vulgatum est." Q. Curtii Rufi, *De rebus gestis Alexandri regis Macedonium,* IX, X, 1.) The question of smallpox in Greek and Roman days has been the subject of debate for the past three hundred years. Certain epidemics have been regarded as due to this infection, but these claims have been hotly denied by other authorities. The only conclusion we can reach at the moment is that we do not know. In Egypt mummies have been found with eruptions resembling those of smallpox and, although one cannot be quite certain, the diagnosis would seem very probable (56).

The earliest undeniable description of smallpox occurring in the West is that of Gregory of Tours, A.D. 580, who gives a detailed account of cases he has seen, followed by that of the Arab physician Rhazes of Bagdad, A.D. 850–932. The latter refers to works of his predecessors on the subject, and there is also a record of the disaster that overtook an Ethiopian army besieging Mecca during the Elephant War of A.D. 569, when 60,000 men died of an illness believed to have been smallpox.

Inoculation against smallpox was introduced into China about A.D. 1000, the method consisting of grinding up the scales and introducing them into the nostril (57), but it took seven centuries before the practice reached Europe via the Greek physicians Timoni and Pylarui, and from there was introduced to England by Lady Mary

Wortley Montagu. This introduction of variolation has been fully discussed by Miller (59).

From this there seems to be little doubt that smallpox has considerable claims to being an urban disease of antiquity.

It will be necessary to consider measles, chickenpox, and rubella together, for they were not clearly distinguished one from the other until the seventeenth and eighteenth centuries (Rolleston). In 1553 a Sicilian physician named Ingrassias (1510–80) wrote a book which was published in Naples, in which he described chickenpox and scarlet fever as being distinct from measles, and this is the earliest accurate record of these infections that has been found. Rubella was described later in the eighteenth century by German physicians, hence its name, "German measles" (57).

There is evidence that measles was present earlier, for the Arab physicians regarded measles and smallpox as different aspects of the same disease. Rhazes gives quite a good description of measles along with his picture of smallpox. Gruner has shown that Europe's first experience with both diseases came in the eighth century during the Saracen invasion, but earlier occurrences are pure guesswork (57). In passing, we may note that the word "measles" first meant leprosy.

Although the evidence is very slight, it is usually assumed that influenza was known in the Mediterranean world during the Greek and Roman empires. Real evidence, however, is not produced until the fourteenth and fifteenth centuries, after which the epidemics were frequent and well-described.

The history of the common cold is very obscure and accurate descriptions of it are not found until modern times.

Mumps are described so well by Hippocrates that there can be no doubt as to its presence in Ancient Greece. "Ardent fevers occurred in a few instances and these very mild, being rarely attended with hemorrhages and never proving fatal. Swellings appeared about the ears in many on either side and in the greatest number on both sides, being unaccompanied by fever so as not to confine the patient to bed; in all cases they disappeared without giving trouble nor did any of them come to suppuration. They were of a lax, large, diffuse character without inflammation or pain and they mostly went away without any critical sign. . . . Many had dry coughs without expectoration and accompanied with hoarseness of voice. In some cases earlier and some cases later, inflammations with pain seized sometimes one of the testicles and sometimes both; some of these cases were accompanied with fever and some were not; the greater part of these were attended with much suffering" (60).

Tuberculosis undoubtedly existed in urban areas in ancient times in the Middle East. Several Egyptian mummies have been found with typical pathological lesions.

Ruffer (1910) states that many of the earlier discoveries are dubious and in some the disease was really non-tuberculous osteoarthritis. There is no doubt, however, that the Egyptians had the disease, and Ruffer has described a priest of Ammon in the twenty-first dynasty, about 1000 B.C., who was buried near Thebes and whose mummy had an unquestionable Pott's deformity as well as a Psoas abscess. The infection seems to have been widespread during the Persian dynasties (525–332 B.C.), but again many of the changes reported may have been non-tuberculous, especially those reported from Macedonian families buried near Alexandria. Wood Jones has described a case which was accepted by Ruffer in which there was reliable evidence of tuberculosis in the spine and elbow. He also reports a case in a small child, possibly dating back to 2700 B.C., which was found by the Hearst Expedition near Gizeh (58).

By the time of Hippocrates, however, from 460–370 B.C., the Greeks were definitely cognizant of pulmonary tuberculosis, and an epidemic appears to have been raging at this time. The description given by Hippocrates is clearcut and easily recognizable: "The greatest and most dangerous disease and one that proved fatal to the greatest number was the consumption. With many people it commenced during the winter and some of these were confined to bed and others bore upon foot; most of these died early in the spring who were confined to bed. Of the others, the cough left not a single person, but it became milder during the summer; during the autumn all these were confined to bed and many of them died, but in the greater number of cases the disease was long protracted. Most of these were suddenly attacked with these diseases, having frequent vigours, often continual and acute fevers, unseasonable copious and cold sweats. . . . The coughs throughout were frequent and sputa copious. . . ."

In Indo-China and China proper the disease is believed to have existed from time beyond memory, being well known to the Annamites under the name of Binh-Ho-Lao, the coughing consumptive disease. Ancient Chinese accounts describe the disease in detail, and records from European missions and physicians report pulmonary tuberculosis ever since Europeans have been present to notice it (60).

There is then good evidence that some of the acute community infections existed in the urban areas before the days of ocean travel. The converse that they did not exist in the non-urban peoples of the world has very little direct data of this kind and what there is is not too definite. For example, with regard to Africa, Cummins quotes Lichtenstein (1803–6) as noting the absence of cough and chronic disease among the Bantu races; Livingstone as having stated in 1857 that among the tribes of the interior "tuberculosis did not exist"; and MacIver, a medical missionary, as adding in 1908 that tuberculosis was not present among the hill peoples in the Shire Highlands in 1894. In 1902 Cummins spent a year with the large but isolated Dinka tribe and found an apparently complete absence of the disease. He quotes the Tuberculosis Commission of South Africa (1914) as stating: "Tuberculosis is of comparative recent introduction among the Bantu races" (61).

However, the reactions of isolated peoples to the infections of Europeans were almost without exception so violent that little doubt can remain after examining the evidence that they were experiencing them for the first time. Some of the data describing this reaction will now be given, starting with the Americas, since they were the largest isolated areas with the biggest populations and the best described epidemics.

The Americas before Columbus were very thinly populated except in the central areas. Various estimates show about eight million people living in territory stretching almost from one Pole to the other. Direct evidence of their infections is very scanty; all records are of chronic infections and not acute ones. For example, as mentioned elsewhere (Chapter 3), lice have been found on the hair of a mummy in the Andes dating back 4,000 years, and whipworm eggs in the intestine of a boy sacrificed and frozen on the top of a mountain in the Andes.

The pre-Columbian Peruvians were skilled at modeling in clay and designed earthenware pots in the shape of men, some showing clearly recognizable infections. Photographs of these have been published by Moodie (1923) and include an achondroplastic dwarf with nodular eruptions of verruga, seated figures removing sandfleas (chigoes) from the feet, and a head with symmetrical bilateral swellings of the nose that resemble "goundoun," treponemal disease. Also depicted are numerous heads with the upper lips cut away as in a disease known as "uta," still extant in those parts and said to be a form of Leishmania (62).

Pinta was mentioned by Cortez in one of his despatches to the Spanish king, in which he described the people as having many-colored patches on their skins. In a recent census in Oaxaca, he says, 12,609 cases of pinta were found among 21,856 people, and many colors of spots on the skin were noted—yellow, red, mulberry, black, lead-colored, mixed white and blue. The American origin of this disease has never been questioned, and this reference by Cortez only serves to confirm it.

Smallpox and measles were taken to Mexico by the Spaniards, and it was epidemics of these, more than any other single factor, that made the invaders' conquest possible. The mortality among the natives from these infections was frightful, but the invaders themselves were not touched, which is a very significant fact from our point of view. Early writers give rather fantastic mortality figures, with the dead running into millions for each infection. Still, there can be no doubt that a large proportion of the population did in fact die from these diseases.

Diaz (63), who witnessed the event, writes:

"Let us return now to Narváez and a Negro he brought with him who was full of smallpox, and a very black dose it was for New Spain, for it was because of him that the whole country was stricken, with a great many deaths. According to what the Indians said, they had never had such a disease, and as they did not understand it, they washed themselves very often, and because of that, a great number of them died, so that black as was the luck of Narváez, still blacker was the death of so many people who were not Christians."

López de Gómara says: "When Narváez' people landed there were among them a Negro with the smallpox which he communicated to the house they had at Cempoallan and then one Indian to another: and as they were so very many and slept and ate together they spread it so much that it went through the land slaying. In most houses everybody died and in many towns the half, as it was quite a new disease for them . . . the Indians called this disease gran leprae. From this, as from a very notable event, they thereafter numbered their years."

The Spaniards were not affected, for they already had had the disease in childhood. So common was it in Spain to suffer from it as a child that Ruy Díaz de Isla remarks, as something unusual, that he knew a man that did not have it until his twentieth year (63).

Similar epidemics followed the invasions of the white people wherever they went. In Peru, there were great outbreaks in 1520,

1533, and 1538, and Pedro de Cieza de Léon said that two hundred thousand Peruvians, including their leader, died in the first wave. In Brazil the 1563 epidemic destroyed thirty thousand natives, and the six colonies established by the Jesuits, and there were other epidemics later. The French took smallpox to Canada with them in the early seventeenth century and, like the Spaniards, were themselves immune. In 1645 the French allies, the Hurons, had a massive infection that changed them from conquering to a weak and defeated nation in flight before the Iroquois. It was the Iroquois' turn next, when a French expedition against them in 1684 failed because both sides had smallpox.

The English settlements were also aided by the disease, and in 1631, according to Mather, "about this time, the Indians began to be quarrelsome touching the Bounds of the land which they had sold to the English, but God ended the controversy by sending the smallpox among the Indians of Sangust, who were before that time exceedingly numerous. Whole towns of them were swept away" (63). Governor Bradford in 1634 describes the pitiful condition of the Indians in a severe epidemic near the Connecticut River settlement and adds, "but by ye marvelous goodness and providens of God not one of ye English was so much sicke or in ye least measure tained by this disease" (64).

Measles spread in the same way as smallpox, the first big epidemic being in 1531, and this disease was called by the Indians *la pequeña leprae,* the "little leprosy." Oviedo and Herrera describe it as very destructive, spreading to Honduras and Nicaragua, then to Peru in 1540. Sigaud said that almost as many Indians of northern and central Brazil died from measles as from smallpox. There were a number of later epidemics, such as that of 1749–50, which killed about thirty thousand people (63).

In Canada the Jesuit Père le Jeune tells of an epidemic among the Indians in 1635 in which the French were also affected but "thank God none died." There was another big epidemic in 1687 (63).

Tuberculosis in the American Indians, it is generally agreed with only a few dissenters such as Mahler, came from the white man. Guthrie said: "Evidence that tuberculosis existed among the Indians prior to the advent of the white man is lacking. Testimony among old Indians would seem to indicate that the disease was seldom seen." The Annual Report of the Canadian Department of Indian Affairs for 1928, quoted by Guthrie, says, "Tuberculosis is about five times more common among Indians than among the general population. Several factors contribute to its prevalence. In many tribes tuberculosis has recently been introduced and the resistance possessed by the white race has not yet been acquired." Unfortunately reliable statistics are very few, especially with regard to the attack and death rate in the tribes before they were placed on reservations or were in close contact with the whites (65).

However, there are many instances of Indian populations in captivity or in reservations succumbing to tuberculosis for the first time. A particularly good example is the imprisonment in Mt. Vernon Barracks in 1887 of several hundred Apaches by the U.S. Government. The tuberculosis death rate rose rapidly, being 54.64 per 1,000 in the first year and 142.83 in the fourth year. The building of new villages and practical sanitary measures notwithstanding, in the fifth year it was still 109.75 per 1,000 and remained about 80 per 1,000 for several years. These figures are said to be reliable, since the Indians were under continuous medical observation (quoted by Ferguson, 1934). These high Indian figures become very significant when compared with the most severe European epidemics, such as that in Belgrade during World War I, when the level of 14 deaths per 1,000 was considered horrifying.

Saskatchewan provides the best data on the progress of tuberculosis among the Indians of the Western Canadian plains. When the buffalo disappeared in 1879, Indians were settled on reservations by the Canadian government and treaty money paid, which meant that a census record was kept. Before that date they had been completely nomadic, almost always in a state of warfare, and had a minimum amount of contact with traders—and, as far as is known, they had little or no tuberculosis. Information on the infection before and after 1879 has been collected by Ferguson (66), who searched the census records for data. The hostile state of these people prevented traders and missionaries from contacting them to any great extent before 1860. A few years after that, infected Indians from Minnesota fled to Canada after a white massacre and about the same time half-breeds, many of them tubercular, were given access to the plains. In 1878 white settlers came in and surrounded the reservations, and soon thereafter Indian children started going to schools.

There had been a number of observers of these Indians in the period from 1800 to 1879, none of whom mentioned cases of tuberculosis, although there had been occasional infections among Hudson's Bay Company personnel. Father Scollen, missionary to the Blackfeet, mentioned smallpox and whisky particularly in a survey

on the decadence of that race, but not tuberculosis; in 1881 he described the recent appearance of the disease in the same Indians.
Ferguson concludes his review of the data before 1879 with the
statement that "it is certain that there were sporadic cases of tuberculosis and equally certain that it was uncommon and unimportant
as a cause of death."

After 1879 it is quite a different story. A most disastrous epidemic
appeared among the tribes settled on the reservations and within
a few years the general death rate among them was varying from
90 to 140 deaths per 1,000, two-thirds of these due to tuberculosis.
The first accurate figures are for 1882, when the epidemic was already under way, the death rate being about 20 per thousand, rising
rapidly to 90 per thousand in 1896, and then gradually subsiding
to about 8 per thousand in the 1930's, which is about 20 times the
rate for the surrounding white population. At first the mortality
was highest in children under 5, though all age groups were heavily
affected, but 30 years later children 10 to 15 years old were most
affected, and there was a marked falling-off in the death rate of
the middle-aged and elderly people. The illness was chiefly the glandular type at the beginning, but over the years this has almost disappeared. In the same Indian school glands were excised in 19.5
per cent of the children in 1905, but in 1921 only 7.4 per cent had
enlarged glands, and in 1932 less than 1 per cent. The reduced death
rate from 1882 to the 1930's was due neither to lack of infection
nor to marked improvement in sanitary conditions, for tuberculin
tests in the 1930's showed that 60 per cent were positive at 7.6 years
and 96 per cent at 11 years. The difference lay in the reaction of the
individual (66, 67).

This severe and prolonged epidemic can be attributed to many
causes: inadequate diet following the disappearance of the buffalo,
poor housing, overcrowding, and general spiritual demoralization.
Yet many Europeans, exposed to conditions as bad as those of the
Indians, do not have mortality figures of this magnitude. In the
first generation all age groups were severely affected, but in later
ones there were fewer deaths among the middle-aged and elderly
groups. All this clearly suggests a new infection spreading among
people not previously exposed to it. Subsequent changes in the character of the disease and reduced death rates in the older age groups
show an increasing resistance, possibly by elimination of the more
susceptible individuals.

The African native is very much more susceptible than the white man, reacting in the so-called "infantile fashion," especially when housed and working in mines and compounds. To quote again from Cummins: "The disease is often of a generalized variety and rapidly fatal, with great liability to vast enlargement of the tracheobronchial glands, caseation, miliary tuberculosis, lesions in the liver, spleen and other organs, and tuberculous pneumonia." This was the type reported by the Transvaal Tuberculosis Research Committee on "Tuberculosis in South Africa natives with special reference to the disease amongst the mine labourers of the Witwatersrand." Roubier in 1920 commented on the differing reactions of Africans from various parts of the continent. Algero-Moroccan troops, who had had

TABLE 6. INCIDENCE OF TUBERCULOSIS IN VARIOUS RACIAL GROUPS

	British Army World War I	
Race	Cases per 10,000	Deaths per 10,000
British and Dominion	6.0	0.4
Portuguese	33.6	9.2
Chinese labor corps	36.3	13.4
Indian troops	93.5	17.2
Indian labor corps	142.0	53.4
South African labor corps	290.0	221.9
Cape Colony labor corps	444.1	103.6

considerable contact with Europeans over long centuries, showed a picture comparable to Europeans, whereas the more isolated and remote Senegalese, as described by Borrel, suffered from the more acute type. African troops were stationed in France after World War I and again the high death rate among the Senegalese troops was very noticeable. In a twelve-month period they had 83.32 cases per 1,000, many being of the acute fatal type, while comparative figures of Mediterranean peoples were: Europeans 9.55, Moroccans 11.73, Arabs 13.33 (61).

A chapter from the Official (British) History of World War I shows the incidence and death rates of various racial constituents from tuberculosis (Table 6). Of course, there were widely differing conditions of hygiene and nutrition, but the variations are so great as to leave no doubt that the Africans reacted much more severely to infection than men from more populous countries (61).

In New Guinea, Heydon (68) found that adult natives from the towns were 29.9 per cent positive to the Von Pirquet test, but only

6.9 per cent of those from the country villages. The town natives had a good deal of contact with the Chinese, who were thought to be very active agents in spreading the infection. Autopsies were done on 29 fatal cases of tuberculosis and, as with the Africans and Indians, it was found that death was due to a very acute and rapidly-spreading form of the disease. Five had lymphatic gland lesions only, 4 tuberculous meningitis, 14 generalized tuberculosis, and only 6 purely thoracic disease.

The Maoris of New Zealand reacted in the same way and the mortality on the east coast, according to Turbott (69), was 49.4 per 10,000, compared with 4.5 for Europeans. Again, variations in environment may account for part, though not all, of that difference.

The Eskimos had no immunity or resistance against the disease. Suk, quoted by Cummins, said: "The prognosis seems hopeless, so strong is the grip of the disease—or rather, so weak is the resisting power of the Eskimo." Tuberculin tests showed that those in close contact with white people on the coasts had high positive rates, for pure Eskimo children were 9.8 per cent positive while the rate among half-castes was 56.2 per cent. A group of visiting representatives of the American Medical Association found that the death rate from tuberculosis in Alaska in 1945 was 359 per 100,000, probably the highest in the world, but that among the Eskimos it was probably 14 times as high as for the whole country. Much of this was undoubtedly due to gross overcrowding in dwellings, where as many as 11 people might be in a room 9 by 12 feet, with very little ventilation. Some, however, may well have been due to racial susceptibility (61).

Australian natives show a similar picture, according to Cleland, Basedow, and other observers (45, 46). Tribes in remote parts of the country had little tuberculosis, but the detribalized natives and half-castes living near missions or otherwise in close contact with whites suffered high mortalities. Clinically, the picture was that described in Negroes, a rapidly-progressing illness characterized by heavy glandular involvement, caseation, and frequently general dissemination of the infection through the entire body.

Perhaps the clearest example of a native community living in a state socially equivalent to that of the hunting era and out of touch with civilization comes from Dutch Guinea. Kahn (70) found a group of bush Negroes living in a most inaccessible part of the country. There were only 18 reactors out of a population of 765 Negroes and 70 Indians. He was able to trace the source of infection to one man who had served as a trader and guide to the coastal area and presumably became infected there. All the positives were in his family; all other families were negative (70).

This picture of introduced infections was repeated in many isolated parts of the world, among the Polynesians and Melanesians of the South Seas, and smallpox among the aborigines of Australia, as we have described in the previous chapter. In the Fiji islands in 1874, when measles was introduced from Sydney, Australia, twenty thousand natives died, although the high mortality here may have been due to the poor quality of native treatment (55). At Rotumah, an island in the South Seas, the mortality was about 21 per cent in 1911, but at Samoa in the same year only 7.4 per cent of the 8,545 cases died, because of the better treatment (55).

It is therefore concluded that isolated areas with small populations did not have the acute community infections until these were introduced from outside. It follows that in other parts of the world these infections could not have evolved until the discovery of agriculture led to increases in population big enough to support them. The acute community infections must have evolved within the past few thousand years.

Theory 6. Agents of these acute crowd infections are derived largely from those of the animals in man's ecology.

As long as he was a wanderer, he could have had very few animals adapted to permanent existence in his ecological habitat, with the exception of the dog, which was mobile and could go with him on his travels. The remainder of the animals he tamed or that came to feed on his camp litter would be left behind when he moved to a new hunting area. In addition, human beings were few in number, and once a group had moved on it would be hard for any animal that had developed a preference for human society to find a replacement. Once man had settled down in villages and towns, many animals would move in beside him—rats and mice, sparrows and pigeons, cats and dogs, goats and sheep, horses and cows, not to mention mosquitoes and ticks—and the pathogens he acquired from them would be passed on from person to person. Once the human population had passed the threshold size, this person-to-person transmission could be maintained indefinitely.

By this continual passage, strains particularly adapted to life in the human host would be selected. Smallpox, measles, mumps, and influenza probably arose this way, certain others may also have done so, and the process is most likely still continuing today. This can be deduced from the fact that the causal agents of these diseases have their nearest relations among pathogens of the animals that live in close contact with man in his ecological habitat. There is the pox group—smallpox in man, vaccinia in cows, infectious ectromelia in mice, fowlpox, swinepox, and other animal poxes; there is the influenza group, containing influenza A, B, and C, mumps, fowl plague, and Newcastle disease, which were grouped together by the New York Conference on Virus and Rickettsial Classification and Nomenclature in 1952; and there are various other groups whose relationship is not yet clearly defined. The poliomyelitis viruses are clearly related to some of those causing encephalomyelitis in mice. The herpes-pseudorabies-B virus groups form an obviously related pattern, and there is also a rather ill-defined group of measles, rinderpest, dog distemper, and swine fever.

These groupings cannot be ascribed to common host phylogenies, as in the case of parasites shared with the primates; and it must therefore be assumed that they represent adaptive radiations of organisms that occupied different hosts, a development that can only have taken place after the hosts came to live together in the same ecological niche—that is, after man settled down.

This transmission of pathogens between the animals within man's ecology is a continuous process and can easily be demonstrated today. Every animal—dog, cat, horse, cow, chicken, duck, rat, mouse, etc.— has some organism to which it is the prime host, but which on occasion spreads to some or all the others in or around the human household. The intestinal organisms usually find it easiest to reach unusual hosts through contamination of food, although modern civilization with its attention to the process, packing, and storing is reducing this risk. Still the ubiquitous rat and mouse are still present in our cities, and in Cincinnati, for example, not a week passes without at least one case of *Salmonella typhimurium* infection being reported. These must originate somewhere in the intestine of one of these rodents. Cats and dogs are perhaps the closest to man in modern civilizations, and both can carry *Salmonellae*. The dog is also the reservoir of *Leptospira canicola,* which is excreted in the urine and numerous cases have been reported where persons handling infectious dogs have developed a meningitis. The first instance of a water-borne outbreak of *L. canicola* infection occurred in Jackson Hole, Wyoming, when 28 boys and girls went swimming together with a dog in a pool fed by a hot spring. Most of them became ill with meningitis due to the dog leptospira (71). Cats have a pneumonitis caused by a member of the psittacosis group and that on occasion is transmitted to children. Hens and ducks have *Salmonellae,* the greatest potentiality for spread of which is through the eggs, especially when these are processed to make dried egg powder.

The dog ascaris sometimes finds its way into children who play in the dirt and swallow the eggs; the larvae hatch out in the unusual host to proceed to a certain degree of development. A heavy infection can be fatal to the child. The cercariae of cow schistosomes can be found in the waters of ponds and streams in many parts of the world, and if the opportunity occurs, they will attack humans. They cannot develop very far, but can cause an unpleasant swimmers' itch as they penetrate the skin. A sheep infection due to a virus called "orf" is well known in the western part of the U.S. and can result in lesions of the hands of sheep herders. Cowpox and bovine tuberculosis, of course, is transmissible to man and even foot-and-mouth disease can occur in man. Birds have salmonellas and ornithosis to contribute to the general interchange of infection, and Newcastle disease can cause conjunctivitis in man. Man himself adds his quota, giving human tuberculosis to his cows to such an extent that it is becoming an increasing problem among cattle raisers to maintain tuberculin-free herds.

These few examples serve to demonstrate that within the group of animals living in man's ecology there is continual exchange of pathogens. The question is which, when, and where will some of these establish themselves in unusual hosts, by being transmitted solely by those hosts and so giving rise to new strains. The difficulty in answering is that the process probably takes a somewhat lengthy period of time for this, and our records are too short for particular examples to become identifiable. Perhaps the best claim is for the influenza virus of the 1918 pandemic. It is now known that when an influenza epidemic sweeps the world, antibodies against the virus can be demonstrated in the blood of many of the animals of man's economy (72). It is also known that hog influenza is due to a strain that is very close to that of man. The very interesting suggestion made is that in 1918 the hogs picked the human strain and continued to pass it within their own populations so that a typical hog strain evolved. Of course the converse is also possible, in that influenza may be basically an animal infection which is sometimes transmitted to man and then spread by continuous human passage.

I have long been intrigued as to the reason why some infections have failed to establish themselves in man. For example, plague, which is primarily a rodent infection spread by fleas, can be spread easily by the airborne route, given the proper conditions, and the pneumonic form of the disease appears in almost all epidemics. Every decade or two, outbreaks of pneumonic plague have appeared during the winter among the tarbagan hunters in the endemic plague area of Manchuria. The most disastrous pandemic of all time was the Black Death, in which it was estimated that one-quarter of the population of Europe died. It seems to have existed in the summer time as a rat infection, but spread from man to man like wildfire in the winter in the pneumonic form that gave it its name. Plague has done this several times, as for instance in the Mediterranean during the reign of Justinian, but always it has burned itself out. Why did it fail to establish itself and to continue as a purely human infection as does measles today?

Another modern example is found in Q fever. The history of this infection is a curious one. Originally isolated from a tick collected near the Rocky Mountain Laboratories, Hamilton, Montana, and identified almost simultaneously as a cause of human disease in Queensland, Australia, it remained as a kind of medical curiosity until World War II. Then suddenly it was found to be the cause of large scale respiratory epidemics in Greece and Italy in 1944–45. The bizarre nature of the ecology of this infection was increased by the discovery of transmission via cows' milk in Los Angeles and the placentas of sheep in Northern California. Obviously this is a widespread zoonosis that has all the potentialities for human adaptation and man-to-man transmission within the human population. Will this pathogen evolve a human strain and continue as has measles, or will it fail to do so as did plague? Only time will tell.

Theory 7. Isolation of a population modifies its infectious diseases.

It is a well-recognized evolutionary theory that isolation of any fraction of a population is the first step toward the formation of a new species, and this is true of both man and his parasites. The isolation may be due to geographical, ecological, or genetic factors.

The example given in this book is a group of infections, the Treponematoses. Since this is described in detail in Chapter 5 on "The Species Concept in Microbiology" and Chapter 7 on "The Treponematoses," no further discussion will be given here.

In brief, the suggestion is made that the natures of the various treponematoses are determined by various isolating factors: Pinta, by being geographically isolated from the rest, while syphilis probably split off from the non-venereal forms about four or five centuries ago when changing habits produced a degree of ecologic isolation. Irkinja in Australia probably evolved originally through geographic isolation, but may have been influenced in the past hundred years by the importation of syphilis.

Theory 8. Some vector-borne infections, such as malaria, originated in the vertebrate.

So far as I can determine, the great majority of workers accept the proposition that arthropod-borne infections originated in the vector and not the vertebrate. Reference to this position has already been made in Chapter 1 in illustrating how a theory should be reversed and tested to see if the converse looks just as likely. In this, mention was made of the work of Hoare (73) and Huff (74), who are strong supporters of the vector origin. However, in reading their papers, I became a little uneasy over some of their arguments and decided to try the opposing theory that some, at least, of the parasites began in the vertebrate. The suggested steps given below for certain protozoa look to me more convincing than those given in the vector-origin theory. They explain why so many cells of the body should be parasitized, and why such diverse types of vectors as leeches, mites, and mosquitoes should be parts of the total picture. The vector-origin theory fails to do this.

An argument usually put forward to support vector origin is that the parasites are better adapted to the vector, and thus must have been associated longer with it. This is not good reasoning. Adaptation of this kind is due basically to natural selection, and the effectiveness of this is not related to time, but first, to the number of generations upon which it acts, and secondly, to the severity of the handicap imposed upon the host by the parasite. When the handicap is severe, the adaptation can proceed to a high degree in only a few generations. The vector has a very short life span compared with the vertebrate. To take an extreme example; the elephant can live until 70 years of age, takes many years to reach maturity, and has a gestation period of 22 months: in this case natural selection and adaptation to a parasite will proceed very slowly as compared to the mosquitoes that feed upon it. A mosquito with several broods a year could develop a high degree of resistance to a parasite in the time it took the elephant to give birth to one offspring.

This theory will be illustrated by the example of malaria and other blood protozoa, whose suggested evolutionary tree will be summarized briefly. We start by assuming that the parasites originated

Table 7. Vertebrate Origin of Certain Vector-borne Blood Protozoa

Suggested paths of evolution.

Primary development in vertebrate

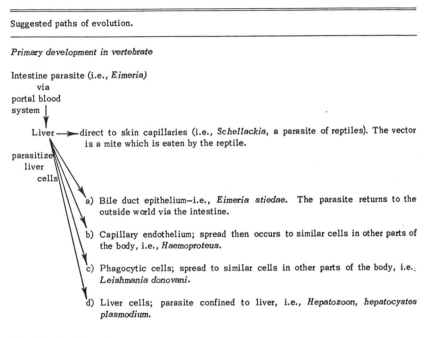

Intestine parasite (i.e., *Eimeria*)
     via
portal blood
system

Liver ⟶ direct to skin capillaries (i.e., *Schellackia*, a parasite of reptiles). The vector is a mite which is eaten by the reptile.

parasitize
   liver
      cells

a) Bile duct epithelium—i.e., *Eimeria stiedae*. The parasite returns to the outside world via the intestine.

b) Capillary endothelium; spread then occurs to similar cells in other parts of the body, i.e., *Haemoproteus*.

c) Phagocytic cells; spread to similar cells in other parts of the body, i.e., *Leishmania donovani*.

d) Liver cells; parasite confined to liver, i.e., *Hepatozoon, hepatocystes plasmodium*.

Secondary developments

a) In the vertebrate; invasion of blood cells which increases chances of transmission, i.e., *Plasmodium, Leucocytozoon*.

b) In the vector; reproduction cycle increasing the number of parasites and thus chances of transmission. *Plasmodium*, etc.

not in the vector's intestine, but in that of the vertebrate. Some would be carried by the portal blood to the liver (75) and in the course of a few million years would parasitize cells there; in the vast majority of cases the process would end with that, for the parasites would be prisoners in their host's body and would die with it. Some, however, would be released from the liver cells into the systemic blood, and of these, a few would be picked up by some of the countless hosts of arthropods that feed every day on vertebrates. Some of the protozoa would be carried mechanically to another host, as happens today with trypanosomes and *Glossina,* thereby initiating the vector-transmission mechanism. Considering the countless number of biting arthropods and the time involved, such a process is almost inevitable. Biting arthropods are known to have existed for hundreds of millions of years, and indeed mosquitoes morphologically indistinguishable from *Culex pipiens* have often been found in Baltic amber thirty million years old (Table 3).

The life cycle of the parasite in the vertebrate would vary according to the type of liver cell involved. Those protozoa that colonized the bile duct epithelium could be excreted to the outside world and reach a new host via the intestine, and thus would not need an invertebrate vector, as is the case with *Eimeria stiedae* (76). The protozoa that colonized cells lining the blood vessels and the phagocytic cells of the liver could spread to similar types of cells in other parts of the body—e.g., *Leishmania donovani,* the agent of kala azar, and *Haemoproteus,* an infection of the capillaries. Those that lived in the true liver cells would of necessity remain there, unless a completely different type of host cell came to be invaded. *Hepatozoon* and *Hepatocystes* are examples of organisms that have remained strictly localized, while *Plasmodium,* the malaria parasite, and *Leucocytozoon,* the blood parasite of birds, are examples of liver cell parasites that can also invade blood cells. This invasion of cells circulating in the blood would obviously be of great help in the spread of a parasite, since it would immensely increase the chances of its being picked up by a biting arthropod and thus passed on to a new host (Table 7). The protozoal infections of the liver have been reviewed by Garnham (77).

Such a concept covers most known facts and avoids many of the inconsistencies inherent in the theory of vector origin. If this is accepted, bird plasmodia, though originating in the same way, would have to be placed in a separate genus from the other plasmodia, since they seem to have parasitized different types of liver cells.

REFERENCES

1. SMITH, T.: *Parasitism and Disease.* Princeton Univ. Press, Princeton, N.J., 1934.
2. ROTHSCHILD, M., AND CLAY, T.: *Fleas, Flukes and Cuckoos.* Philosophical Library, New York, 1952.

3. SONNEBORN, T. M.: The cytoplasm in heredity. Heredity, 1950, **4:** 11–36.
4. BISSETT, K. A.: Characters associated with parasitism in gram positive bacteria. Nature, 1959, **184:** B.A. 29.
5. WARDLE, R. A. AND McLEOD, J. A.: *The Zoology of Tapeworms.* Univ. of Minnesota Press, Minneapolis, 1952.
6. CAMERON, THOMAS W. M.: Animal parasites & human diseases. Proc. N.Y. Acad. Sciences, 1958, **70:** 564–73.
7. ANONYMOUS: First Symposium on Host Specificity among Parasites of Vertebrates. Inst. Zool., Neuchâtel Univ., Neuchâtel, Switzerland, 1957.
8. HUXLEY, J.: *Evolution.* Harper & Bros., New York, 1942.
9. FERRIS, G. F.: The sucking lice. Pacific Coast Entom. Soc., N.Y. Lithographing Corp., New York, 1951.
10. HOPKINS, G. H. E.: "The Distribution of Phthiraptera on Mammals." *In:* Symposium on Host Specificity among Parasites of Vertebrates. Inst. Zool., Neuchâtel Univ., Neuchâtel, Switzerland, 1957.
11. PATTERSON, B.: Mammalian phylogeny. *In:* Symposium on Host Specificity among Parasites of Vertebrates, p. 26 (see above).
12. WEBB, J. E.: Phylogenetic relationships of the anoplura. Proc. Zool. Soc., London, 1946, **116:** 49–119.
13. WARRINGTON YORKE AND MAPLESTONE, P. A.: *The Nematode Parasites of Vertebrates.* Blakiston, Son & Co., Philadelphia, 1926.
14. CAMERON, T. W. M.: *Parasites & Parasitism.* John Wiley & Sons, N.Y., 1956.
15. DOBELL, C.: Amoebae of monkeys. Annual Report, Med. Res. Counc. Rep., 1924–25, pp. 31–33.
16. DOBELL, C.: Intestinal protozoa of monkeys. Annual Report, Med. Res. Counc. Rep., 1926, pp. 35–36.
17. HEGNER, R.: The protozoa of wild monkeys. Science, 1929, **70:** 539–40.
18. HEGNER, R. AND CHU, H. J.: Protozoal infections of 44 wild Philippine monkeys. Amer. J. Hyg., 1939, **12:** 62.
19. KESSEL, J. F.: Experimental transfer of intestinal protozoa from man to monkeys. Proc. Soc. Exp. Biol. & Med., 1924, **22:** 206–8.
20. KESSEL, J. F.: The dysentery amoeba of monkey and man. Proc. Soc. Exp. Biol. & Med., 1926, **23:** 675–76.
21. KESSEL, J. F.: Intestinal protozoa of monkeys. J. Parasit., 1927, **13:** 283–84.
22. KESSEL, J. F.: Intestinal protozoa of monkeys. Univ. Calif. Pub. Zool., 1928, **31:** 275–306.
23. ABERLE, S. D.: *Primate malaria.* Nat. Res. Council Washington, D.C., 1945.
24. BRUMPT, E.: *In:* Boyd, M. F., Ed., *Malariology.* W. B. Saunders Co., Philadelphia, 1949.
25. CHRISTOPHERS, R.: Malaria from a zoological point of view. Proc. Roy. Soc. Med., 1934, **27:** 991–1000.
26. KEBLE, S. A., CHRISTOFINIS, G. J., AND WOOD, W.: Natural virus B infection in rhesus monkeys. J. Path. & Bact., 1958, **76:** 189–99.
27. HILLIS, W. D.: Infectious hepatitis from chimpanzees. Amer. J. Hyg., 1961, **73:** 316.
28. HUEBNER, R. J.: Personal communication. 1958.
29. BOYD, M. F.: *Malariology.* W. B. Saunders Co., Philadelphia, 1949.
30. WEBSTER, L. T.: Experimental epidemiology. Medicine, 1932, **11:** 321.
31. WEBSTER, L. T.: Experimental epidemiology. Medicine, 1946, **25:** 77.
32. TOPLEY, W. W. C.: The biology of epidemics. Proc. Roy. Soc. Med., London, s. B, 1942, **130:** 337.
33. GREENWOOD, M., HILL, A. B., TOPLEY, W. W. C., AND WILSON, J.: Experimental epidemiology. Med. Res. Council, Special Reports Series 209, London, 1936.
34. SABIN, A. B.: Nature of inherited resistance to viruses. Proc. Nat. Acad. Sci., 1952, **38:** 540–46.

35. FENNER, F.: Myxomatosis. Brit. Med. Bull., 1959, **15**: 240–45.
36. ANDREWES, C. H.: The effect on virulence of changes in the parasite and host. In *Virus and Virulence*. Ciba Foundation, Little, Brown & Co., Boston, 1960.
37. ALLISON, A. C.: Malaria and sickle-cell anaemia. Brit. Med. J., 1954, **1**: 290.
38. FERGUSON, R. C.: A study of tuberculosis among Indians. Trans. Amer. Clin. & Climat. Assoc., 1934, pp. 1-9.
39. FERGUSON, R. G.: Tuberculosis among the Indians of the Great Canadian Plains. Trans. 14th Ann. Conf. Nat. Assoc. Prev. Tuberc., Adlard and Son, Ltd., London, 1934.
40. STRODE, G. K.: *Yellow Fever*. McGraw-Hill Book Co., New York, 1951.
41. ASHBURN, P. M.: *The Ranks of Death*. Coward-McCann. New York, 1947.
42. McCULLOUGH, F. S.: The distribution of *Schistosoma haematobium* by Bilinus sp. in the Ke District of the Gold Coast. Trans. Roy. Soc. Trop. Med. & Hyg., 1956, **50**: 449–57.
43. PANUM, P. L.: Measles in the Faroe Islands. Delta Omega Society, New York, Amer. Pub. Health Assoc., 1940.
44. BODIAN, D.: Emerging concepts of poliomyelitis infection. Science, 1955, **122**: 105–8.
45. CLELAND, J. B.: Disease among the Australian Aborigine. J. Trop. Med. & Hyg., 1928, **31**: 53–59, 66–70, 141–45, 157–60, 173–77.
46. BASEDOW, H.: Diseases of the Australian Aborigines. J. Trop. Med. & Hyg., 1932, **35**: 177.
47. MANN, I.: Possible origins of trachoma in Australasia. Bull. W.H.O., 1957, **16**: 1165–87.
48. MANN, I.: Personal Communication.
49. JELLIFFE, D. B., WOODBURN, J., BENNETT, F. J., AND JELLIFFE, E. F. P.: The children of the Hadza hunters. Trop. Paed., 1962, **60**: 907–13.
50. BATES, M.: Population as a unit of study. Cold Spring Harbor Symp. Quant. Biol., 1950, **15**: 36.
51. BEDSON, S. P., DOWNIE, A. W., MacCALLUM, F. O., AND STUART HARRIS, C. H.: *Virus and Rickettsial Diseases*. Edward Arnold Publisher, Ltd., London, 1955.
52. CHURCHILL, W. S.: *History of the English-Speaking Peoples*. Vol. *1*, Cassell & Sons, Ltd., London, 1955.
53. MEANS, P. A.: *Ancient Civilization of the Andes*. Charles Scribner & Sons. New York, 1942.
54. MOONEY, J.: *Aboriginal Population of America*. Smithsonian Misc. Coll. no. 7, Smithsonian Institution, Washington, D.C., 1928.
55. HIRSCH, A.: Handbook of Geographic & Historical Pathology. The New Sydenham Society, London, Vol. I, *Acute Infectious Disease*. Trans. from 2nd German Edition, 1883.
56. RUFFER, SIR M. A. AND FERGUSON, A. R.: Smallpox in a Egyptian mummy. J. Path. & Bact., 1911, **15**.
57. ROLLESTON, J. D.: *History of the Acute Exanthemata*. Heineman, London, 1937.
58. RUFFER, SIR MARC ARMAND: *Studies in Palaeopathology of Egypt*. Univ. of Chicago Press, Chicago, 1921.
59. MILLER, G.: *The Adoption of Inoculation for Smallpox in England and France*. Univ. of Penn. Press, Philadelphia, 1957.
60. HIPPOCRATES: *Genuine Works of Hippocrates*. Translated from the Greek by Francis Adams. Wood, New York, 1849, p. 366.
61. CUMMINS, S. L.: *Primitive Tuberculosis*. John Bale Medical Publication, London, 1939.
62. MOODIE, R. L.: *The Antiquity of Disease*. Univ. of Chicago Press, Chicago, 1923, p. 148.
63. STEARN, E. W., AND STEARN, A. E.: *The Effect of Smallpox on the Destiny of the Amerindian*, Bruce Humphreys, Boston, 1945.

64. Bradford's History "Of Plimoth Plantation" from the original manuscript. Commonwealth of Mass., Wright & Potter Printing Co., Boston, 1928.
65. GUTHRIE, G. M.: The Health of the American Indian. Public Health Rep., 1929, 44: 945.
66. FERGUSON, R. G.: Tuberculosis among the Indians of the Great Canadian Plains. Trans. 14th Ann. Conf. Nat. Assoc. Prev. Tuberc., 1934.
67. FERGUSON, R. G.: A study of tuberculosis among Indians. Trans. Amer. Clin. & Climat. Assoc., 1934, 1–9.
68. HEYDON, G. M.: Tuberculosis of the territory of New Guinea. Med. J. Aust., 1924, 18: 277.
69. TURBOTT, H. B.: *Tuberculosis in the Maori*. Department of Health, Wellington, New Zealand, 1935.
70. KAHN, M. C.: Tuberculosis of the bush Negroes of Dutch Guiana. Amer. Rev. Tuberc., 1937, 35: 36–40.
71. COCKBURN, T. A., VAVRA, J. D., SPENCER, S. S., DANN, J. R., PETERSON, L. J., AND RHEINHARD, K. R.: Human Leptospirosis associated with a swimming pool. Amer. J. Hyg., 1954, 60: 1–7.
72. MEENAN, P. N., BOYD, M. R. AND MULLANEY, R.: Human influenza viruses in domesticated animals. Brit. Med. J., July 14, 1962, pp. 86–90.
73. HOARE, C. A.: The relationships of the haemo flagellates. Proc. 4th Int. Cong. on Trop. Med. & Malaria, Washington, 1948.
74. HUFF, C. G.: Studies on the evolution of some disease-forming organisms. Quart. Rev. Biol., 1938, 13: 196–206.
75. WENYON, C. M.: *Protozoology*. Wood, New York, 1926.
76. SMETANA, K.: Coccidiosis of the liver of rabbits. Arch. Path., 1933, 15: 516–36.
77. GARNHAM, P. C. C.: The liver in relation to protozoal infections. Proc. Roy. Soc. Trop. Med. & Hyg., 1949, 43: 649–58.

CHAPTER 5

The Species Concept
In Microbiology

IN MICROBIOLOGY, ideas as to what constitutes a species are still largely typological in nature, a concept which in zoology and botany has been abandoned to a considerable degree. Most biologists now would agree to some variation of the definition of a species as being "a population of interbreeding or potentially interbreeding organisms that is reproductively isolated from all other such populations." This definition can be expressed in many ways, but the two essential points are the interbreeding and the isolation. So long as microorganisms were considered to reproduce by some means of asexual fission, such a definition was simply not acceptable. This situation has changed dramatically with the discoveries of conjugation, transduction, and transformation involving bacteria and viruses, so now it is becoming increasingly clear that genetic materials are in fact shared among individual microbes. As a result, the population concept of a species must be applied to microbes as well as larger creatures. There can be no hypothetical threshold of size, on one side of which the larger creatures have species' units of one kind, and on the other, the smaller ones have quite a different kind. Both must have the same. Providing the isolating mechanisms can be demonstrated, the concept of a species as an isolated interbreeding population is not difficult to visualize among the protozoa where sexual forms of organisms such as *Plasmodium* and *Paramecium* have been well studied; nor among the bacteria, where the existence of the various forms of genetic exchange of conjugation, transduction, and transformation have been described in some detail. The main trouble starts with the viruses, for although the exchange of genetic materials between individual virus particles is established without doubt, there is considerable uncertainty about their very nature. Should they be regarded as genuine organismal bodies, or merely parts of other organisms, or even are they dead or alive? To me, the question of being dead or alive is merely a matter of semantics. If, as it seems, the forms of activity which we call life are dependent solely on the presence of certain compounds containing nucleic acids, then there is a continuous sequence of chemo-physical states ranging from the simplest chemical to the most highly developed creature. There is no abrupt transition from one stage to another; therefore, there is no point on the scale at which one of these can be called alive and the next with a few less atoms is not alive. The division of all matter and energy into living and dead must be an artificial one created by man, and does not exist in reality.

In investigations into matters such as the nature of virus, a working hypothesis can be a useful device, and this personal one is therefore offered for what it is worth, and without any attempt being made to justify it. In this, the essential part of the virus is the RNA. Under primitive earth conditions, simple precursor forms of this must have existed in the oceans, in discrete particles bathed in solutions of hydrocarbons and amino acids. Some particles would break up and their components would be incorporated in others, thereby causing a constant state of interchange of substances. Those particles, which by chance had acquired the more efficient catalysts, would grow in size and complexity at the expense of those without them: this process of interchange of materials and catalysts would be of prime importance in the origin of "life." This would be of value later in the evolution of higher forms, with the catalysts now elevated to the status of enzymes. The simplest forms of exchange—that of breakdown and incorporation into other particles—would have survived to the present day in the process of transformation. On a larger scale, the union of two complete particles drawn together by the possession of unlike electric charges would be even more efficient; at this level, the particles would be somewhat of the dimensions and organization of "free-living" viruses and this would be the origin of transduction. Later, as the oceans' supplies of building materials became exhausted, being concentrated in the particles, some of the larger particles would evolve their own microclimates in the nature of cytoplasm-containing envelopes that would approximate to some extent the conditions in the oceans of the primitive earth. This, however, would lead to difficulties in the transfer of substances between one organism and another. The simpler methods of transformation and transduction would still be of value and would continue in spite of the evolution of sexual means of exchange. In this working hypothesis, many viruses are therefore separate and distinct entities, although very simple in nature; in most cases they would play an important part in the survival of the cells with cytoplasm with which they are associated, although some that have gone astray in one way or another cause damage, and these are the ones we recognize as pathogens.

In the course of the hundreds of millions of years since the origin of "life," many cells that had been engulfed by larger ones must have been preadapted to life within the bodies of the others, and so came to parasitize them. As first suggested by Laidlaw (1), these parasites would in time lose the enzyme systems that would be surplus within the host cell and in time would degenerate into virus-like creatures. These however would not necessarily benefit the host cell by any mechanism of gene transfer, but would be entirely parasitic. Therefore, there might well be two kinds of viruses, the older kind living in a kind of mutualistic state with the cells except for a few that have developed pathogenic tendencies, and the more recent types that are basically parasites. So far as the species concepts are concerned, both kinds would be individual organisms that can properly be considered for species rank.

The classification of bacteria and viruses has of course been discussed many times in works of taxonomy, at various Congresses of Microbiology, and a symposium was held by the New York Academy of Sciences in 1952 (2). A recent paper by Ravin has been a big step forward (3). Probably most microbiologists would agree with Andrewes when he said that "systems of nomenclature are for man's convenience and cannot hope to be wholly logical as to represent faithfully the evolutions of all living things" (4). Those who believe that the species is a distinct natural entity that would exist whether or not man was there to study it are in a marked minority and the proponents of a natural system of classification are few in number. In recent times, Kluyver and van Niel have proposed a system based upon evolutionary concepts (5), and this was supported by Stanier and van Niel who said that there is good reason to prefer an admittedly imperfect natural system to a purely empirical one (6). However, at a symposium in New York in 1952, almost all speakers were in favor of the purely empirical approach, although Waksman came close to the population concept of a species by emphasizing that the range of variation must be established before a species can be claimed, and that minor variations or even certain qualitative variations from descriptions of recognized species are not enough.*

---

* The 12th Symposium on Microbial Classification recently published for the Society of General Microbiology (Cambridge University Press, 1962) serves to reveal the utter

The 1950's have seen big strides made in the understanding of bacterial and viral genetics, and by 1954, the effect of this on concepts of speciation could be seen in the papers presented at a meeting of the Society for General Microbiology in September of that year on the principles of microbial classification. Whereas at the New York Symposium of only two years earlier there had been little or no attempt to use the population concept of a species, by the time of this later meeting, several speakers indicated an interest in it. The most notable was Pontecorvo who discussed the impact of genetics on microbial classification (7). To him, a species in higher forms of life is "an aggregate of individuals which, directly or indirectly, can contribute over an indefinite number of generations to a common pool of hereditary determinants." "There is great individual variation within a species and to distinguish individuals of one species from those of a closely related one we use the yardstick of gene flow versus gene isolation. I hasten to repeat that even in the systematics of higher organisms this criterion is barely beginning to be used, and that for a long time in many groups it will have to be used only as an inference." Now as to microorganisms, I repeat that the systematics of no group is as yet ripe for the "impact."

Since 1954, microbiologic genetics has continued its amazing progress, but it will be a long time before a microbial classification can be set up based entirely upon a population concept of a species and the yardstick of gene flow and gene isolation. Still, there is enough knowledge now to attempt some visualization of the process, and that is attempted in a general way in this chapter. No effort will be made to review the literature on genetics, for such works are already in existence and the paper by Ravin (3) gives an excellent account of much of the application of this to the species concept. The main effort here will be a discussion on the second factor, gene isolation and its relationship to the species and classification.

confusion prevailing on the concept of a species. Some of the contributors had doubts as to the existence of a natural species, and one went so far as to title his paper "The Microbial Species—A Macromyth?". Nowhere in the symposium was there any support for the population concept given in this present book. It seemed agreed that microbes, on present knowledge, cannot be arranged in a hierarchical system to show their phylogeny. The position today is, in fact, something much like that of biology about the time of Linneus, with creatures being arranged into species on the basis of similarity and without regard to ideas of populations or evolution. In my opinion, this is only a phase through which microbiology will pass. Most of the groups chosen by similarity will prove to be natural populations for the reason that organisms of any kind that interbreed tend to be more alike than those that do not.

The Typological Concept of a Species

According to Simpson (8), the basic concept of typology is this: "every natural group of organisms, hence every natural taxon in classification, has an invariant generalized or idealized pattern shared by all members of the group. Variations within the species, the "accidents" of the scholastics, are a nuisance but (or because) they have no taxonomic significance." "On typological principles any specimen of a species embodies its 'type' and hence is adequate for defining the species and as a standard of comparison."

The typological concept is the only one possible when a new field of biology is being opened up, as when the new flora and fauna of Australia were first being brought back to Europe, or when tissue culture reveals new kinds of viruses in respiratory and intestinal tracts. A type specimen is set up and all new finds are compared with it. The trouble starts when increasing numbers of specimens are collected, numerous variants are found, too many species are named, and a battle then starts between the "splitters" and the "lumpers." Let us illustrate the process utilizing the hypothetical man from Mars, who is visiting the Earth collecting strange birds. While visiting Washington, he shoots a white pigeon, takes it back to Mars, and describes a new species. He is followed by another Martian who collects a brown one and a blue one, compares them with the type specimen, and describes two new species on the basis of the color. Soon large numbers of specimens arrive on Mars, and variations other than that of color are discovered and more new species described until it seems there will be as many species as specimens of pigeons. At this stage, the "lumpers" get busy, and insist on only a few species based on color; unfortunately many pigeons are bicolored or even multicolored, but these are dismissed as being atypical and everyone tries to forget them. Then some live pigeons are taken to Mars, and it is found that if two pigeons of different colors are mated, the offspring may have both the colors or even sometimes have a third color. At this confusing stage, a physiologist finds that the birds have blood groups and claims that the blood group antigens are more basic and natural than colors for classification and sets up a completely new serologic system. Of course, this means changing all the names, but it is argued that they have all been changed a dozen times already, so what does once more matter.

In the modern world of microbiology, for "pigeon" read *Salmonella*, respiratory virus, enterovirus, cancer virus, etc.

A good example of the typological concept as used by the hypothetical Martian can be seen today in the enteroviruses. The first of these to be discovered was polio virus, and this was isolated in 1909 from neural tissue (9). By 1912, the virus had been recovered from the feces (10), but it was some decades before the connection with the intestinal tract was firmly established (11). By that time, another series of intestinal viruses, the Coxsackie group, were being revealed by a technical advance in the use of baby mice. Soon there were three polio viruses and two groups of Coxsackie virus, with 6 types in group A and 23 in group B. The development of tissue culture methods in the latter 1950's led to the recognition of other enteroviruses, the presence of which had been unknown, and which had no obvious connection with any disease. These were called the ECHO viruses, and quickly 28 different types were described and numbered. However, type 10 proved to be much larger than the others and to have typical cytoplasmic inclusions, and was placed in a new "Reo" group of which there are now three members.

As data accumulated, it was found that not only did intermediate forms exist, but that there was considerable overlapping of characters from one group to another, so that some of the ECHO viruses will cause Coxsackie-like pathologies in mice, while Coxsackie ones will produce cytophathogenic effects in tissue culture. A type A Coxsackie virus will cause paralysis in monkeys and has been called Type 4 polio virus by the Russians. The next step has been to call a conference at which it was voted to abandon all these names and group all the viruses together and just give them serial numbers. Already in the animal field, related or parallel viruses are being recovered, and, presumably in the future, some attempt will be made to include these in the classification. But not until an arrangement is made, based upon units existing in nature and ordered according to their evolutionary history, will stability and the maximum utility be obtained in the classification of the enteroviruses.

This typological approach is inevitable in the early stages of discovery for there is no alternative to the method, but carried to a conclusion it can result in confusions of various kinds. This is well demonstrated by the example of the genus *Salmonella*. The first members of this genus were discovered in the early days of bacteriology and the early steps were very much like those of enteric viruses of today. The bacilli were first described by their shape and staining reactions; later, the ability to ferment various sugars was used to differentiate the various species; then as animal infections were discovered, the organisms were given names according to the animal host, such as *typhimurium* and *cholera suis*. As data accumulated, strains of *Salmonella* were discovered that had atypical sugar fermentation reactions, while the various animal types were isolated from hosts other than those named. Finally the antigenic method was adopted, and this has proved of considerable practical value for many years. However, as more data were acquired, difficulties have arisen again, for every new combination of antigens in the bacillus has been placed in a separate group and by now, there are over 800 of these "species." Most workers avoid the name of species by calling them "serotypes," but still use the binomial nomenclature usually reserved for species, and use these groupings as though they are, in fact, just that. The list is growing at the rate of about 50 a year, and it has been calculated that the total number of permutations and combinations of the various antigens allows for many thousands of possible "species." Already the number is rendering the scheme increasingly cumbersome to use, but that would not be of serious import if the "species" were stable and genuine. Unfortunately, in the laboratory it has proved possible to change many of the "species" into other "species," either by conjugations of two organisms of different "species" (12) by transmission of genes by phage (13) or by growing the organisms in appropriate sera (14). Apparently, the antigenic components of the bacterial cell are not much more reliable as specific characters than are the sugar reactions, morphology, or any other such indicators. The typological approach to classification is the only means available in the early stages of discovery, but is inadequate where fuller information is at hand.

The Adansonian variant of the typologic form of classification is of importance because of its recent use in bacteriology by Sneath and his followers (15, 16). In this, as in most systems, there is the underlying assumption that there is a natural order, a system of similarities, which can be discovered by investigation. The groupings themselves would be artifacts of man, so that the species itself would not really exist in nature. "God can consider every creature as an individual—we have to group them into things as species and genera. Only creatures exist" (Adanson, 1763). In each group, the overall similarity is measured by the number of similar features, each feature having an equal weight in measuring overall similarity.

The operative word is number; the overall similarity is the concept of sharing many features and not only one. No one feature is regarded as more important than the other, and as many as possible are considered.

Applying this concept to bacteriology, Sneath has described a method for handling large quantities of taxonomic data by an electric computer so as to yield the outline of a classification based on equally weighted features. This enables *similarity* to be expressed numerically and would allow taxonomic rank to be measured in terms of it. The method is to count the number of similar and dissimilar features between strains and to sort into groups those with a high percentage of similarities. A similar system of groupings has been suggested by a number of workers in general biology, including Michener and Sokal (17), and the pros and cons of this have been reviewed by Simpson. Simpson (8) raises two objections, the first being that many of the features fed into the computer may have resemblances due to homoplasy and not homology. In homoplasy, the resemblances are the result of parallelism, mimicry, convergence, analogy, or chance, whereas in homology they are due to the common ancestry that is the basis of most modern classifications. Using large numbers of characters probably does tend to reduce the effect of homoplasy on the result, but some effect is always possible and it may be so great as to invalidate the result. Second, it is spurious to think that using multiple characters increases probability if the characters are closely correlated either genetically or functionally. Characters that are perfectly or highly associated certainly should not be considered independent items of evidence, but only as one item.

The attempts to use the computer as a tool in classification are very interesting, but only time will tell if they will be successful. Certainly, in measuring the variation within a species population, a system based on a computer might be well worth-while. However, in defining the species as a whole and its relationship to others and where a phylogenetic system is to be erected, the search must still be for characters that are basic in evolutionary development. The difficulty is that there is no good rule for deciding exactly which character is old and which is recent in appearance. This will be discussed later.

The Concept of the Isolated Population

The definition offered here is as follows: "A species in the fields of protozoology, bacteriology, and virology, is a population of organisms within which genetic determinants are exchanged by transformation, transduction, or any other means, and which in Nature has been isolated from spread of such determinants from all other populations for time enough to permit the evolution of distinct and measurable variations from all other populations." *

Such a definition is too abstract to be of use in everyday routine work, for in innumerable laboratories in all countries, everyday names have to be given to newly isolated organisms. This practical need can be met by research workers first outlining the range of variation within the specific population as well as the extent of its distribution, and then choosing a comprehensive series of morphological or biochemical markers that can be identified in a practicing laboratory. A relatively simple range of markers covering most variations could be provided for a hospital laboratory, a more complex one for a reference laboratory of the stature of a state laboratory, while a specialist working on a particular group of organisms would have to be familiar with the complete range of variation.

The definition given above is one of perfection that will be difficult to realize at present. It will take a long time to gather all the information required to decide the varying degrees of genetic homology between organisms and the boundaries of the breeding populations. Regardless of this, one feels that the time to begin thinking on these lines has now arrived, and suggestions as to how the matter might be tackled is given later in this chapter with the *Salmonellae*. A fuller attempt at defining the limits of a species is given in the account on the origin of the treponematoses in a later chapter.

---

* It must be realized that all parasitic organisms, to a large extent, are isolated in the host in which they live. A single bacterium can infect a man and within a few days grow into a population of countless millions of individuals. These will be isolated from all other similar populations unless a second infection of the host takes place. Of these countless millions of individuals, all will die either with the host or when the host resistance increases beyond a certain threshold point. Only a very few lucky individuals will be successful in invading a fresh susceptible host and thus starting the process all over again. However, mixed infections will occur and this will permit the exchange of genetic material between the bacteria infecting the various hosts.

Isolation in Speciation

Without isolation of breeding populations, the species of today could not have been created. If during the period of time that life has been on earth there had been no obstacles to prevent the interchange of hereditary determinants between creatures, then all would have been much alike. Whenever a new determinant arose it would quickly have been shared by all the creatures on earth, so that all would have much the same forms and characteristics. It is only when prevention of such sharing arises by one mechanism or another that variations can be produced by the accumulation of mutations or unusual groupings of hereditary determinants in the isolated populations.

Geographic isolation was obviously a very great factor one or two thousand years ago, before the ocean-going vessel was developed; the exchange of microorganisms from one continent to another must have been a rare event, apart from those carried by the wind or seas, migratory birds, bats, or fishes. The chances of a streptococcus or treponeme being carried from Australia to Europe or from America to Africa would be extremely remote, until man came along to aid in the transport. In the chapter on the origin of the treponematoses, it has been theorized that the pinta of Central America evolved there as a result of such isolation. The treponemes were probably carried there by man in his wanderings around the world, and must always have experienced some isolation merely due to distance, but when the Ice Age ended and the rising seas cut off America from Asia at the Bering Straits, this must have become almost complete.

Other differences in infections between America and the rest of the world included the apparent absence of smallpox and measles from the New World in the days before Columbus, and the existence of forms of trypanosomal and leishmanial infections peculiar to that continent. In the final chapter of this book, it is suggested that malaria is a recent import. Yellow fever was probably also absent until introduced by ship from West Africa (18). *The Salmonellae* of the New World are known to differ substantially from those of the Old World, as was vividly demonstrated in the late war when the isolation broke down. Huge quantities of dried egg were imported into England as an emergency measure, and this was heavily contaminated with *Salmonellae*. In the 17 prewar years 1923–39, only 14 different species of *Salmonella* had been identified as being responsible for food poisoning in Great Britain, with never more than 7 species in one year, and all being well-recognized European ones. The shipments of dried egg began in the latter half of 1942, and by the end of the year no fewer than 18 species were identified in outbreaks and, of these, 10 were American species never previously isolated in Great Britain. By 1944, 24 new species had been introduced to Great Britain from the New World (19). With the ending of the war, the shipments of dried egg were largely halted, *Salmonellae* no longer crossed the Atlantic in such quantity.

Ecologic Isolation

Related organisms may occupy an area that is undivided geographically yet may be isolated from one another by some feature of behavior or transmission. Possibly syphilis and yaws arose in this way from one common infection as described in Chapter 7. The treponemes causing these diseases are morphologically much the same, and there is considerable cross immunity between the two infections. There is no geographic barrier to prevent either infection occupying the territory of the other, yet syphilis is not common in the endemic yaws areas of the tropics, while yaws is rare in the temperate areas of syphilis. The explanation given is that the treponeme is a very delicate organism that cannot survive long away from its host, so that almost direct contact between persons is necessary for transmission. In the tropics where few clothes are worn, a treponeme on any part of the body has a chance of reaching a new host and so surviving, but in colder climates where people cover most of their bodies to keep warm, only treponemes that are transmitted during the sexual act have a fair chance of surviving. A syphilis treponeme arriving in an endemic yaws area is at a biologic disadvantage, since much of the population there will be immune before puberty is reached. In this fashion, two forms of treponemal infection will exist side by side without geographical separation.

Of course, all vector-borne infections are limited by the distributions of the vector. All zoonoses are limited in distribution by the ranges of their prime hosts. Many infections have climatic requirements, so that malaria is not found in cold climates, although anophelines are abundant there.

Host isolation results from a high degree of host-parasite adaptation, which in turn must often be dependent upon the method of transmission available to the parasite. Where the means of transfer to new hosts is direct, as in the skin-to-skin spread of the scabies acarus, lice, or yaws treponemes, or venereal as in syphilis or the trypanosomal infection of horses, the new host found by the parasite is likely to be of the same species as the former. This form of passage will inevitably result in a parasite that is so highly adapted to its host species that it will be unable to live in other hosts. Speciation in this form of parasite will be in step with that of its host, as described in other parts of this book.

Sex isolation occurs where individuals of two species fail to interbreed because of inability to complete the mating act. Such difficulties are well known in the larger parasites like fleas and helminths, the sex organs of which are sometimes so highly specialized that these characteristics are used by taxonomists in classification at the species level. In recent years, it has been discovered that bacterial recombination is dependent on a factor F^+ without which mating will not take place. The factor has not been isolated in an extracellular form but after infection of the bacterium acts as though an addition to the genome. It may be either unintegrated or fully integrated; in the latter form as in Hfr bacteria that have a high frequency rate of recombination, the factor is incapable of infecting other bacteria while permitting mating with them. This factor F^+ may permit mating with some recipient bacteria and not others, and perhaps one bacterium may have two separate F^+ factors. Two bacteria that are unable to mate with one another may each mate with a third, so that in a large population of bacteria, there may be small groups of bacteria that are to a large degree similar to one another but cannot mate, yet may not be in complete isolation, since genetic exchange may occur through the agency of a third group of organisms that conjugates with both.

Genetic isolation in its various degrees depends upon the extent of genetic homology between two bacterial populations. This field has been reviewed recently by Ravin (3) from whose paper the following examples are taken. When differences occur, the genetic exchange may be incomplete in spite of high frequencies of success in bacterial combinations, phage infection, or transformation with DNA. For example, there is high frequency of conjugation between *Shigella* F^- and *Escherichia coli* F^+, which may come as high as between two strains of *E. coli* F^- and F^+, yet the rate of genetic recombination is substantially lower. It has been argued that this is the result of the incompleteness of the genetic homology between *Shigella* and *Escherichia*.

In transduction by phage, isolation is encountered in that usually the phage is specific for only the one species of bacteria. However, mutants that infect other species may arise, or sometimes a phage will infect a number of organisms that taxonomists of the typologic school place in more than one species. For example that phage PLT 22 derived from a lysogenic strain of *Salmonella typhimurium* can bring about antigenic recombination between other strains given taxonomic status. Several serotypes can be produced, some of which are known to exist in nature and some that have not been recognized as yet. Should phage PLT 22 function in this manner in nature, then the strains of *Salmonella* involved in the genetic transfer would all have to be classed as belonging to one species, and not several as would be the case if the proposal of Kauffman were accepted that each organism with a distinctive antigenic structure be given specific rank.

Transformation, the spread of genetic material by DNA, is becoming increasingly recognized as a factor of considerable importance. The DNA that is liberated from autolysing cells in a culture can be as effective as that extracted by chemical means, as has been demonstrated in the interspecific transformation of *Neisseria* species. Here again isolation occurs to a considerable extent, since a barrier to spread by this means is the requirement of a degree of genetic homology for the process to be a success. However, as in recombination and transduction, some transformations take place between organisms placed in different species, as between *Haemophilus influenzae* and *H. parainfluenzae* and also between two strains of *Streptococcus viridans* and *S. salivarius* or pneumococci. Apparently, full transformation occurs only with exact pairing of the DNA form in the donor and recipient; in hetero-specific transformation, integrated markers might be freed from those adjacent regions of the exogenous molecule that causes lower probability of integration.

Partial Isolation

Probably no large population is completely homogenous in the sense that the exchange of genetic material between the individuals in it is totally free and unhampered. This would only be achieved if the environment were completely uniform and the distances were not so great that mere space alone would not slow down the drift of determinants from one edge of the area to the other. Usually in any territory there are localized environmental variations that produce natural selection pressures peculiar to themselves and these are reflected in the populations of creatures living there. Any hindrance in the flow of determinants in or out of these small pockets will accentuate these differences, producing a partially isolated variant population called a "deme." The isolating mechanisms can be any of those described earlier. Partial isolation of this kind may be responsible for much or even most of the atypical or variant strains of organisms that are commonplace in all fields of microbiology and parasitology. Every protozoologist, bacteriologist, or virologist is familiar with variations of this kind, whether it be the *Plasmodium* with unusual morphology, the bacterial strain that does not ferment the "right" sugars, or the virus with the unusual host range or cytopathogenic effects. In the population concept of a species, these are not "atypical" organisms, but merely part of the normal variation that is to be found with the population that is a species.

Some organisms appear at first sight to have only one species with little or no variation within it, and rabies virus is a classical example of this. Yet, on closer examination, the presence of demes and the variations they produce can be seen there also. One deme in the rabies virus population is found in the bat hosts; the mechanisms by which the virus is maintained within the non-vampire bats are not yet known, although it is likely that spread can take place from the bats to other animals that eat the dead or dying bats or are attacked by sick bats or by aerosols in bat caves. Undoubtedly, the bat virus is partially isolated from that of other animals and the variations that result from this are demonstrated in two ways. First, the incubation period of bat virus in test animals is longer than that derived from other mammals, and secondly, the inclusion bodies are much smaller. When the usual stains are used, the Negri bodies so typical of dog rabies may not be seen in the bat type, but the use of the fluorescent antibody technique reveals their presence as very fine dust-like particles.

Universal Populations

Some organisms are spread throughout the world and infect many kinds of animals, and yet show little in the way of variation. Typical of these is rabies virus mentioned above, and also *Salmonella typhimurium* and the plague bacillus, *Pasteurella pestis*. Influenza virus can cover the human populations in an amazingly fast fashion, and during a pandemic of influenza, virus isolants made from all parts of the world are very similar to one another. All these organisms have two characteristics in common; they all are capable of crossing geographic barriers and have methods of transmission that scatter the individual organismal particles throughout many parts of the animal world. Rabies virus is carried by migrating bats; plague and *S. typhimurium* are basically infections of the ubiquitous rodents; influenza is transported everywhere by man, and scattered widespread by airborne droplets. The spread of rabies virus to all mammals is ensured by the biting of carnivores or sick non-carnivorous animals, plague by the biting of infected fleas that become hungry after their host dies and therefore are liable to attack almost any animal, while *S. typhimurium* in the feces of rats and mice is ideally placed to contaminate any foodstuff or water. These organisms therefore have no difficulty in traveling almost anywhere and infecting many animals, so that isolation for them is unlikely. During influenza pandemics, very little variation can be detected in the strains of virus isolated from various parts of the world, and this is possibly due to the rapid exchange of infections from one part of the world to another. Later in the pandemic, the growing immunity of the peoples of the different countries will hamper this spread and also eventually cause the pandemic to disappear, so that pockets of infection will replace the earlier generalized condition. These pockets will in fact be partially isolated populations of virus or demes, and may tend to give rise to variant strains of virus.

Peripheral Populations

The organisms in the center of the ecological niche occupied by the species receive genetic exchanges from all sides, while those on the periphery, where conditions are marginal and natural selection pressures most severe, are recipients from one side only. These peripheral ones will be prevented from full adaptation to the severe conditions in their area by these arriving determinants from the center that are less adapted to the severe conditions. Should they be cut off completely from the main population, they will quickly evolve into a new species. However, conditions may be so extreme that the peripheral population may not survive unless reinforced by new arrivals.

The process can be illustrated with the arbor viruses. Western Equine arbor virus is basically an infection of birds transmitted by a mosquito, *Culex tarsalis*. This mosquito has a preference for birds' blood, but obtains a percentage of its feeds from mammals. During the summer periods in endemic areas, the virus spills out from the bird-mosquito cycle so that almost any mammal can be infected, including man, horse, and a wide variety of small mammals (20). In the mammals so far tested, the titres of virus produced in the blood have been found to be usually too low to infect possible vectors and so permit the establishment of further mammal-mosquito cycles, although possibly in substantial epizootics, this may happen to a small degree. Any bloodsucking arthropod feeding on a bird or mammal with virus in its blood may have its biting mouth parts infected or take a sample of the virus into its stomach; indeed, many isolations of virus have been made from such arthropods, including the wild bird mite *Dermanyssus americana,* the chicken mite *D. gallinae, Triatoma,* and species of mosquitoes not thought to be part of the regular bird-mosquito cycle. Most of the lives of these peripheral viral populations in mammals and accidental insect infections will be very brief, disappearing unless reinforced from the main bird-mosquito reservoir. Some will be longer lasting if the infected mammals produce enough virus in their bloods to infect the mosquitoes feeding on them; but with only rare exceptions will a peripheral infection of this sort survive the adverse conditions that come with the onset of cold weather. Occasionally, it is possible that this rare event will take place, and when it does, a few passages of the virus in the new host and vector may produce a strain of virus better suited to that particular cycle. It is probably in this fashion that there evolved the wide range of arbor viruses that are being discovered all over the world.

Classification and the Species Concept

In everyday routine in laboratory or field study, the microbiologist is constantly faced with the problem of giving a name to some organism, and he needs some easy and quick way for doing this. He requires some combination of characters that are definite, specific, and unchanging that will apply to one classification unit only, this unit being also definite, specific, and unchanging. Academically, he is asking for the impossible; for all life is under constant change, and in microbiology, new strains of organisms may appear almost overnight, as happens with influenza virus or drug-resistant forms of bacteria and protozoa, but in practice, a way has to be found to help him.

The principle of classification expounded here is a natural system derived from the phylogeny of organisms, the foundation of such a system being the species. The higher echelons recapitulate the past history of the species, so that it follows that all the species in one genus are descended from one common ancestor and all the genera in one family similarly have a common descent, and so on. The problem of the taxonomist is to work out the steps of this evolution for each kind of organism, and then having arranged the fundamental relationships and circumscribed the limits of the species, to look for characters that will cover as far as possible the range of variation within that species. It may not be possible to find characters that will do this and not overlap with those of other species, but in routine practice an approximation may be adequate for the purpose.

In using the population concept of a species, always it must be remembered that a character in itself does not make a species, but is merely a guide to finding the population to which the organism in question belongs. It is not enough to have one type specimen as a standard for comparison of all unknowns; the range of variation must be explored and a selection of type specimens maintained for comparison purposes. These type specimens must indicate all the forms in which the particular character can be expected to be found. Any kind of character can be used with advantage, and except for convenience in handling and as described later, there is no reason why any one kind of character should be chosen over another. All of them, from the morphologic, physiologic, behavioral, to the antigenic, are equally affected by inheritance, mutation, and natural selection, and so liable to change, although it is a general rule in biology that those which are thought to be oldest phylogenetically prove to be the most suited for classification purposes. Size and shape are usually useful, but there are many environments in which these become grossly distorted; staining reactions, capsule formation, sugar fermentation, effects on test animals or in tissue culture are all unreliable and subject to variation according to the prevailing conditions.

An increasing tendency is to use antigenic characters for classification, and the process has gone so far that Kauffmann has proposed that all *Salmonella* organisms with different antigenic patterns should be given specific status (21). This reflects unbiologic thinking, for an antigen is no more reliable than any other character and indeed is only a reflection of some character in the body of an organism. The antibody production is a function of the creature invaded by a parasite. Through the antigen-antibody reaction we are able to measure conveniently an array of substances in the parasite, but these substances are no more than ordinary characters of that parasite, and in the great majority of cases, they have not been identified, so we do not know what we are measuring. For example in *Salmonella* the various antigens have been represented by various numerals and letters, but what these mean in the body of the bacillus is not known. Since we do not know what they are, often we cannot tell if the substances they represent are old phylogenetically or of recent origin; what is quite clear is that they are simply the physical characters reflected in a form that can be easily identified and measured. They may be in the flagellum, cell wall, enzyme system, or nucleus, but wherever they are, they are subject to the same forces as any other part of the organism.

"Convergent evolution" is the process in which a number of different species occupy the same environment, are therefore subject to many of the same pressures of natural selection, and come to have certain superficial resemblances. For example, the whale which is a mammal and the shark which is a fish both live in the sea and have superficial resemblances. Both have become streamlined by having the same need for moving through the water as quickly as possible. The whale is thought to have been descended from a bear-like land animal that took to the water, but now looks much like the shark. Similarly all microorganisms living in the same place superficially look alike. All bacteria that live in hot springs are similar in that they must be able to survive temperatures that are higher than usual, those that parasitize man have an optimum temperature range about 37 degrees centigrade, while those living in soil and surface water grow best at a lower temperature. Most creatures living permanently in fluids, excepting viruses, have some means of progressing through those fluids, and the choice is restricted to a limited range of forms, including a twisting rotation that often results in a spiral shape, or the evolution of flagella or undulant membranes. Those exposed at some time to life on dry land must have adaptations to avoid dessication, and again this is largely limited to spore or cyst formation or thickened walls. Features such as these are adaptations of a convergent nature to a common environment, and the sharing of such by microorganisms does not of itself reflect phylogenetic relationships.

An organism that has proceeded through the stages from a free-living form to that of a parasite has obviously undergone a series of adaptions to new environments that will be reflected in the characters used for classification. Some of these changes will be due to convergent evolution and be common to all parasites within the prevailing environment, and it would be a mistake to group the organisms by these secondary adaptations. The suggestion has been made that the universally used Gram positive or negative character is one of these. Gram positivity is now thought to be the result of the possession by the bacterium of a high molecular complex, formed by combination of reduced basic protein substrate with magnesium ribonucleate. Experimentally, this complex can be removed and later restored again with corresponding alterations in the Gram's stain (22). According to Bisset (23), the loss of the Gram positive reaction is possibly associated with the availability of complex nutrients, so that here is a tendency for highly adapted parasites to be Gram negative. Other adaptations to parasitic life that apply to all microorganisms include the change from aerobiosis to anaerobiosis and a progressive loss of structures and functions that are no longer essential under the new conditions. Among the examples given by Bisset is the genus *Neisseria,* all the members of which are clearly related by morphology, metabolism, and antibiotic sensitivity, but where the facultative parasitic members are Gram positive and the obligate parasites are Gram negative. Often a series of forms can be demonstrated linking a Gram positive aerobic complex saprophyte with a Gram negative anaerobic parasite of simple morphology. Such a linkage is seen between the *Sarcinae* equipped with flagellum and spore, the Gram positive micrococci and staphylococci without the flagellum and spore, the Gram negative or variable members of *Neisseria,* and in turn the anaerobic, Gram negative, and very small bacteria of the species of *Veillonella.*

The same kind of linkage from saprophyte to parasite is found in *Mycobacterium.* The genus is based upon the characters of acid-fastness, absence of flagella and motility, reproduction by simple binary fission, and absence of spore formation, but none of these properties are constant and all vary continually. The parasitic strains are said to have certain distinct properties, such as limited temperate range, pathogenicity, formation of "serpentine cords," niacin synthesis, and specific cytochemical reactions, but Xalabarder (24) has pointed out that most of these are in reality biologic deficiencies and has listed twenty-three metabolic functions of saprophytes that are missing in the pathogenic organisms. These range from the ability to utilize creatin, urea, and air as sources of nitrogen, sixteen chemicals as the source of carbon, to growth in the presence of copper and silver, and the reduction of methylene blue and dichloro-phenol. Nor is pathogenicity a unique characteristic, for pathogenic strains can easily be converted into non-pathogens, while the reverse process can be achieved by growing saprophytes in filtrates from virulent strains.

It is convenient at times to talk about the respiratory viruses, the enteric bacillae, enteroviruses, or the encephalitis group of arbor viruses, but such terms should not be confused with a classification based on phylogenetic principles. They can properly be used only in the sense as the animals of South Africa, Australia, or the fishes of the sea. Just as the whale who lives in the sea is descended from a land animal, a parasitic bacterium or virus may have resulted from the spread of the infection from some totally different creature. (Basically, it is regarded as axiomatic that all parasites are derived from free-living forms.) Very often it must happen that the nearest relation to a parasite is not some other one in the same host, but rather a parasite in some other host.

Parasites are sometimes grouped according to the vectors that transmit them, and this again can be misleading, for an arthropod-borne agent may be closely related to one without a vector. An example of this is found in the genus *Trypanosoma*, most of the species of which are insect transmitted. However, one species, *T. equiperdum*, has extended its geographic area to places where suitable vectors are lacking by adopting the venereal method of spread. It is, in fact, surprising that more vector-borne infections have not succeeded in doing this, for many of them can spread readily without their vectors if the circumstances are suitable. Plague, for example, readily becomes a respiratory infection in winter and where overcrowding is prevalent, while tularemia epidemics on a large scale can be caused by infecting the water of streams in which infected muskrats are living and dying. On the other hand, it is surprising that the bed-bug has not been found to be a vector of some human infection.

The problem of deciding if any particular group of organisms forms a species resolves itself into two questions: first, do all strains in the group have enough genetic homology to permit major exchanges, and secondly, is there ample opportunity for free exchange of genetic material without any isolation, beyond those partial and peripheral kinds described earlier? If these conditions prevail, then until shown otherwise, all members of the group must be considered as one species. The genetic homology can be demonstrated by conjugation, transduction, and transformation experiments; degrees of isolation can be detected by field studies of the ecology of the infections with regard to geography, host range, means of transmission, and vectors, if any. Once the ranges of genetic variation and general ecology of a species have been determined, all newly discovered strains that fall within those ranges will automatically be considered as belonging to that species.

It is not practical for the average worker in a busy laboratory to undertake all the steps outlined above, so to help him, a range of characters must be chosen that will represent the main features and variations of the individuals within the species population. These must be easily recognizable and will act as a short cut to identification of the appropriate population. However, they are unlikely to cover all the variations within the species population and, perhaps it might be possible to produce identification keys with varying degrees of accuracy; for routine purposes one with 80 per cent coverage of variation could be provided, another with 95 per cent probability, and for the specialist, there would be a complete list of the variations. It is at this level that the use of the computer would be valuable. The single type specimen would be supported with a collection of specimens representing the entire species population.

Once the population that is the species has been defined by combined laboratory and field studies, and the range of variation within it has been clearly outlined, perhaps with the assistance of a computer, the next step is to look for characters or markers for use both in deciding the relationship with other species and for everyday utility for identification in the practicing laboratory. This is the most difficult task in biology and it can be said immediately that no "golden rules" exist to help in the matter. The general statement usually made is that those features which are the oldest phylogenetically are usually the best and most stable, but that only poses the question as to how those features can be distinguished from the more recent ones. There is no simple way of doing this, so the studies must include the relationship of individual characters to the organism as a whole, and the organism in relation to its own ecology, as well as other species that are related or competing, or apparently similar. The terms "primitive" and "specialized" are used for characters within a taxon, being relative to one another and dependent in proportion to their departure from the ancestral condition. Some guidance on the search for primitive and specialized characters has been given by Simpson for larger creatures (8), and these can be adapted with advantage for microorganisms. It must be emphasized that none of these are without exceptions, but they are of some value.

First, "in contemporaneous sequences, more primitive characters will be those that have evolved more slowly," and will be less likely to change now in response to minor variations in ecology. For instance, mycobacteria are grouped to a large extent on their property of acidfastness, although many organisms can be found that are not acid fast at times in their life cycle and possibly all mycobacteria produce forms that do not possess the characteristic (25). Another character that is of value is that of virulence, but virulence for any given test animal is a very labile affair in comparison to the comparative steadiness of the acidfastness reaction, and must therefore be considered as more recently specialized and less primitive than the other. To convert a non-pathogenic commensal *Mycobacterium* to a virulent form without the use of genetic material from such an existing form is probably difficult and time consuming, while it is easy to select strains non-pathogenic to the usual test animals from those that are pathogenic.

Secondly, characteristics that are more general in nature are likely to be more primitive. The difficulty is that general ones are usually shared by many different forms which have acquired these characters by convergent evolution and not homology. However, when a species invades a new environment, it will have not only the adaptions to the new environmental conditions but also considerable inherited features reflecting the influence of a former environment. For example, the mammals that entered the sea to live wholly there, now have a superficial resemblance to fishes, but still retain the basic bony structure of their limbs. Sharks have never walked on dry land and so do not have vestigial limbs. Applying this to the vibrios, both parasite and non-parasite, it is obvious that these are organisms that have been adapted to an aquatic existence for a very long time, perhaps for as long as there have been bacteria in existence. They are found in waters in all parts of the world, and some have become commensals or parasites of other creatures such as fish and various mammals including man. Wherever found, they show all the features of creatures highly adapted to the aquatic environment and none of those of the dry land. In the open water, speed is apparently of great value for survival, and a single propellant at the rear is very efficient. Organisms with multiple propellants along the body, like legs or cilia, may do well on land or in certain fluid situations, but in open water, these are not efficient. Just as the whale has dispensed with its four limbs and now has a single tail at the rear, so the flagella of the vibrios are very few in number and at the rear. The vibrio has none of the features needed for life in a dry environment, for it has no spore, no cyst, no thick-walled forms, and soon dies out of water. Morphologically, the most outstanding feature is its comma shape, although many other forms are found, especially in old cultures. This comma shape probably has an advantage for a rapidly moving organism in that it will travel to some extent in a circular fashion, and therefore not out shoot an area where conditions and food are favorable, while still being able to move out from unfavorable circumstances. This adaptation to a total fluid existence must be a very primitive one. Characteristics such as these would, of course, evolve in any organism living in a similar environment, so that those now classed as vibrios may represent several different groups. Yet numerous vibrios from many parts of the world have so many other features in common, including antigens and transduction by common phages, that most may be descendants from a common ancestral species. The virulences of pathogenic vibrios of man and domestic animals must be recent specializations, geologically speaking, judging by the rapidity with which the pathogenic vibrios revert on culture to non-pathogenic forms.

Thirdly, "intricate functionally coordinated structures are less liable to close convergence, and an aspect of that fact is that they tend to be less labile and to retain ancestral conditions longer. The ear region in mammals is such a structure, characteristically with delicate coadaptation among its parts. It is probably in all such cases that there is a correspondingly complex and delicate coadaptation in the genetic substrata. Almost any change then requires difficult changes throughout the complex and will be rejected or only slowly coadapted by natural selection." In microbes, this will apply to all complex metabolic systems, whereby the food taken in is broken down by a series of steps, each requiring an enzyme reaction, and then utilized by another series of reactions. The more complicated the procedure, the more difficult it will be for evolutionary forces to alter it, and therefore such complex metabolic systems can be regarded as comparatively primitive and of value in classification. In the early days of bacteriology, sugar fermentation was given a leading role in the identification of certain bacteria, and indeed the method still has a good place in the laboratory. Yet, sugars require only comparatively simple metabolic mechanisms for their utilization, and therefore are subject to rapid evolutionary change. This reduces their value from the point of classification.

Fourthly, "the most conclusive evidence as to primitive (and hence ancestral) characters is provided when one condition in a group or one end of a sequence has a homologue in another group of more remote ancestry." For example, the platypus, the kangaroo, and man are all classed together as mammals, but the platypus lays an egg and this is a reptilian feature, so that its mode of reproduction is regarded as more primitive than those of the other two. Similarly, when the reproduction of bacteria is studied, and the larger viral type agents such as those of the psittacosis group and the smaller viruses are compared, it is seen that the small viruses reproduce by a process that more nearly resembles that of straight DNA replication, and indeed, they can do this even though lacking all other parts except their DNA. Therefore, this method of reproduction must be more primitive than that of the others which proceed through a more complex cycle.

Loss of a character by mutation and natural selection is a common event. In any phylogenetic tree, all the descendants of the original ancestor had of course in the beginning all the characters of that ancestor, but in the course of time some would lose various ones of these. For example, all mammals and reptiles are thought to have originated from an ancestor with five toes, for none of them have more than five toes, though many have less. The five-toed condition is regarded as being more primitive than the one toe, which is regarded as highly specialized. (It cannot be argued, however, that because the horse has lost four toes and now only has one, and the cow has lost only three toes, that the one toe of the horse is more primitive than the two toes of the cow.) Similarly, in bacteria, those that have the full range of enzyme systems for metabolizing a particular substance must be more primitive than those that have lost the means of completing certain steps and therefore have to depend upon finding the missing substances or "vitamins" in the environment. Bacteria that have acquired an intracellular form of life find many of these essential requirements inside of the parasitized cell, so that when mutants lacking certain enzymes do arise, natural selection may not operate against them and they may survive. In this way, parasitic bacteria will tend to lose characters, so that the absence of many enzymes, as indicated by high nutritional requirements, is more likely to be a recent specialized feature as compared to the more primitive condition where all are present and the organism is capable of living on simple nutrients.

All these guidelines are useful in helping to arrive at a decision as to which character is primitive and which is a recent specialization, but often they are quite inadequate. In general, there is no sub-

stitute for a total study of the related organisms and their environments. When this is done, often most difficulties resolve themselves.

Let us apply this process to the genus *Salmonella*. Probably all
members of the genus have the same general genetic framework, but
individual species might have peculiarities that would be susceptible
to analysis. Already much work has been done on these lines, so
that many of the present "species" or serotypes are known to be con-
vertible into others, as described earlier. Two organisms that can
interchange successfully most of their genetic material are potential
members of the same species. Those that cannot do this do not belong
to the same species.

Geographic isolation of *Salmonella* groups will often be fairly
obvious in a general way. Organisms that are native to a continent,
and not obvious recent imports, are likely to differ from those of
other continents, so that, for example, a whole range of *Salmonellae*
exist in the Americas, belonging to populations isolated from those
in Europe, and many could be given specific rank because of this.
The exceptions to this rule will be those *Salmonellae* of migratory
birds, fish, and bats or animals that have no difficulty in traveling like
some small rodents, cockroaches, or domestic pets.

Salmonellae that are largely confined to one species of animal are
likely to be isolated populations, and worthy of specific rank. Examples would be *Salmonella typhi, cholera suis, typhi suis, pullorum,
gallinarum, dublin, abortus, equi,* and *abortus ovis,* for although
these are all found from time to time in other animals, these exceptional ones are in the nature of peripheral populations. Should the
infection in the main host disappear, in time those in the exceptional
hosts would soon follow suit.

Some species will be of the universal type described earlier, such
as *S. typhi murium,* which is basically an infection of rodents associated with man, and as such liable to gain access to all parts of
the world and many species of animal host.

In this way it would be possible to describe a relatively small number of species, all to a large degree isolated from each other, and all
capable of interchange of genetic material between individuals within
the population. There would be considerable variation within each
population, so that new species would not be claimed merely because
a strain of *Salmonella* was recovered from an unusual host, had a
peculiar sugar reaction, or some unusual combination of antigens.

The method of antigenic analysis could be retained for general
use in *Salmonella* studies, for it is a convenient tool, and much data

has been accumulated. Within each species a range of antigenic variation would be described so that the mere absence of one antigen or the presence of an extra one would not by itself be of undue significance, although it might lead to further studies on the ecology of that particular strain.

In fields like the enteroviruses or respiratory viruses, the process of isolating new strains, comparing them with other known ones, and then giving arbitrary names will have to continue until enough data has been amassed for a critical review. The data needed would include details of related viruses from many forms of animal host besides that of man, for in many instances, the nearest relations of the human ones are likely to be found in other animals.

REFERENCES

1. LAIDLAW, P. P.: *Virus Diseases and Viruses.* Cambridge Univ. Press, Cambridge, 1938.
2. NEW YORK ACADEMY OF SCIENCES: Virus and rickettsial classification and nomenclature. Ann. N.Y. Acad. Sci., March 31, 1953.
3. RAVIN, A. W.: The origin of bacterial species. Bact. Rev., 1960, 24: 220.
4. ANDREWES, C. H.: Viruses and Linnaeus. Acta Path. Microbiol. Scand., 1951, 28: 211–25.
5. KLUYVER, A. J. AND VAN NEIL, C. B.: Prospects for a natural classification of bacteria. Bakt. (Abst. 2), 1936, 94: 369–403.
6. STANIER, R. Y. AND VAN NIEL, C. B.: The main outlines of bacterial classification. J. Bact., 1941, 42: 437–66.
7. PONTECORVO, G.: Principles of microbial classification. J. Gen. Microbiol., 1955, 12: 314–86.
8. SIMPSON, G. G.: *Principles of Animal Taxonomy.* Columbia Univ. Press, New York, 1961.
9. LANDSTEINER, K. AND LEVADITI, C.: Transmission of acute poliomyelitis to monkeys. Compt. Rend. Acad. d. Sci., 1909, 149: 1014.
10. FLEXNER, S., CLARK, P. F. AND DOCHEZ, A. R.: Experimental poliomyelitis in monkeys. J.A.M.A., 1912, 59: 273.
11. BODIAN, D.: Emerging concepts of poliomyelitis infection. Science, 1955, 122: 105–8.
12. ZINDER, N.: Sexuality and mating in *Salmonella.* Science, 1960, 131: 9124–26.
13. LEDERBERGER, J.: Genetic transduction. Amer. Scientist, 1956, 44: 264–80.
14. TAYLOR, J.: Why christen a salmonella? Int. Bull. Bact. Nomen. & Taxonomy, 1959, 9: 159–64.
15. SNEATH, P. H. A.: Some thoughts on bacterial classification. J. Gen. Microbiol., 1957, 17: 184–200.
16. SNEATH, P. H. A.: The applications of computers to taxonomy. J. Gen. Microbiol., 1957, 17: 201–26.
17. MICHENER, C. D. AND SOKAL, R. S.: A quantitative approach to a problem in classification. Evolution, 1957, 11: 130–62.
18. CARTER, H. R.: *Yellow Fever, an Epidemiological and Historic Study of Its Place of Origin.* Williams & Wilkins, Baltimore, 1931.

19. Medical Research Council Special Report Series No. 260: The bacteriology of spray-dried egg. H.M. Stationery Office, London, 1947.
20. COCKBURN, T. A., SOOTER, C. A. AND LANGMUIR, A. D.: The ecology of western equine encephalomyelitis virus in Colorado. Amer. J. Hyg., 1957, 65: 130–46.
21. KAUFFMANN, F.: Der Bakteriologie der Salmonella sp. Einar Munksgaard, Copenhagen, 1961.
22. HENRY, M. AND STACEY, M.: Histochemistry of the gram staining. Nature, 1943, 151: 671.
23. BISSET, K. A.: Characters associated with parasitism in gram positive bacteria. Nature, 1959, 184: B.A. 29.
24. XALABARDER, C.: The so-called problem of unclassified mycobacteria. Amer. J. Reps. Dis., 1961, 83: 1–15.

CHAPTER 6

The Basic Principles
of Eradication

"ERADICATION" OF INFECTIOUS disease as a concept in public health has been advanced only within the past two decades, yet it is replacing "control" as an objective. The meaning of the term varies with the user, and the difficulties of achieving eradication, in any form, are usually underestimated.

My own definition of eradication was published in 1961 (1) and received a wide acceptance in public health circles in this country. As a result of this article, a seminar on the subject was held at the annual meeting of the American Public Health Association in Detroit, November 1961, and again there was substantial agreement with the idea I had expressed, although there were some who had reservations. By chance, the following day, a similar seminar, confined to tuberculosis, debated the same principle. Here, however, some of the tuberculosis workers on the panel would not agree to the "total" concept as expounded by Dr. Fred L. Soper, the invited speaker, but insisted that eradication meant the elimination of the disease as a public health problem. Therefore, the mere presence of a few cases did not mean that the target had not been hit (2).

In this chapter my own definition of eradication is offered; the difficulties common to all schemes of eradication are discussed; and the significance of animal parasites in this connection is outlined.

Definition

In my definition, eradication is the extinction of the pathogen that causes the infectious disease in question; so long as a single member of the species survives, then eradication has not been accomplished. The definition implies action on a world-wide scale, but world-wide eradication has not yet been achieved for any infection.

"Regional eradication" implies a basically unstable situation, because at any time the infection may be reintroduced by carriers or vectors from outside. The occurrence of occasional small episodes of infection in a cleared area does not invalidate the claim that regional eradication has been achieved in that area, provided the infection was imported.

For areas where vectors are present but without the parasite, one may still claim eradication—as, for example, in Sardinia where there are anopheles without the *Plasmodium,* and in the United States where there are *Aedes aegypti* without the yellow-fever virus. In South America, yellow-fever virus cannot be eradicated, since it is endemic in the monkey population of the forest; however, eradication of the domestic vector *A. aegypti* from the continent is under way, and this situation could be defined as "urban" eradication of yellow fever, and "regional" eradication of the mosquito.

Even if world-wide eradication of an infection is achieved, there is the possibility that a similar infection may evolve from related organisms still existing in nature after measures of eradication have been halted.

There is an essential difference between the concepts of eradication and control. Once eradication is achieved, the infection is gone forever, and the costly burden of recurring control measures may be dropped. Eradication can, therefore, be regarded as that state in which the infection does not return from infected areas after control measures have been abandoned. If procedures have to be continued to prevent return of the infection, then the state is one of control and not eradication.

Some pathogens persist in the body for long periods of time, and, strictly speaking, eradication has not been accomplished until the last parasite has died. However, in regional eradication, the practical definition can be used, and each infection can be judged independently. For example, in Brill's disease the rickettsiae persist in the body for very many years; in the United States, there must be people who became infected abroad and who are still carrying the pathogen, yet the infection must not be regarded as established here, since the chances of transmission are remote. Similarly, in malaria, the parasite can persist in the body for years; many people in the United States are infected, but because the likelihood of transmission is very small, even without control measures, eradication can be claimed. The situation is different in an area where conditions favor the transmission of malaria; should eradication measures based on mosquito control be abandoned while the parasite still persists in the human host, then, even though the disease has not been reported for some time, there is a possibility of a recurrence of transmission, and the claim of eradication is not justified.

In world eradication programs, the strictest adherence to the definition should be maintained; thus, in the case of smallpox virus, which can live for many months on infected clothing, a time allowance on this scale should be made after all other signs of the infection have disappeared. In malaria, before eradication as defined here can be claimed, there must be many years' surveillance after the last case has been diagnosed.

The definition given above is in general agreement with the World Health Organization's definition for malaria eradication. In its original form the World Health Organization's definition (3) was interpreted as meaning "the ending of the transmission of malaria and the elimination of the reservoir of infective cases in a campaign limited in time and carried to such a degree of perfection that, when it comes to an end, there is no resumption of transmission." The criteria of malaria eradication to be adopted included adequately demonstrated absence of transmission and endemicity for a period of at least three years, in at least the last two of which no specific general measures of anopheline control and no routine chemotherapy had been applied (4). The World Health Organization's definition was modified still further to give more precision to the surveillance requirements (5), but it still does not go so far as to include the final elimination of the last parasite and does not mention related infections in animals or the theoretical possibility that the infection may evolve again.

History

Deliberate attempts to stamp out infectious diseases began in the closing years of the last century. In 1892, an animal infection, contagious pleuro-pneumonia of cattle, was declared eradicated from the United States after a campaign that lasted five years and cost nearly two million dollars (6).

In England, in 1896, rabies was eradicated successfully by enforcing a muzzling order for all dogs for one year and enforcing a three months' quarantine for all dogs and cats at their owner's house. In 1901, a fresh order imposed a period of six months' quarantine in premises under control of a Veterinary Surgeon. This was reduced to four months in 1914 and extended again to six months in 1918.

The results of these measures was the number of cases of rabies in dogs dropped from 151 in 1897 to 2 in 1902 and none thereafter until 1918. The quarantine system was not totally effective during the later stages of World War I and an epizootic resulted. In 1918 there were 98 cases and the following year 150; but only one in 1922 and no more in unquarantined dogs since that time to the present. The last instance of the disease in a quarantined dog was in 1949 (7).

In 1917, the decision was made to eradicate bovine tuberculosis in the United States, under the Federal-State Cooperative Plan for Eradication of Bovine Tuberculosis. The program called for the testing of all cattle in the United States and the killing of the reactors, and it was extremely costly both in money and in animals. The campaign was not pushed to the extreme required for eradication, and it was unsuccessful in that bovine tuberculosis still exists in this country (6). Yellow fever was eliminated from Cuba in the first decade of this century by anti-mosquito measures, and this gave rise to such high hopes that in 1914 Gorgas could state that world eradication of the disease not only was practical but could be achieved at a reasonable cost (8). With the discovery of forest yellow fever, these hopes were disappointed and the idea of eradication was discredited.

Modern ideas on eradication begin with the work of Soper and his colleagues in South America. In 1930, some dangerous African mosquitoes, *Anopheles gambiae,* were discovered in Brazil by Shannon, and in a few years these had spread and were the vectors responsible for a disastrous epidemic of malaria in the northeast section of the country. A program to eradicate every single specimen was begun in 1939, and by 1941 the task had been completed (9). Side by side with this program, the control of *Aedes aegypti* mosquitoes had progressed so well that in 1942 Soper was encouraged to propose eradication instead of control. The following year, Bolivia was the first country to proclaim that this goal had been reached. Since that time the countries of South America have joined forces, aiming for complete continental eradication. By 1960, substantial areas had been cleared (10) (Figure 5).

These successes with mosquito eradication made eradication a respectable term once more, so that world eradication of smallpox and malaria are now proclaimed aims of the World Health Organization, in programs supported by many countries and backed financially by the United States. At present, eradication is described as the aim in many other infectious-disease projects.

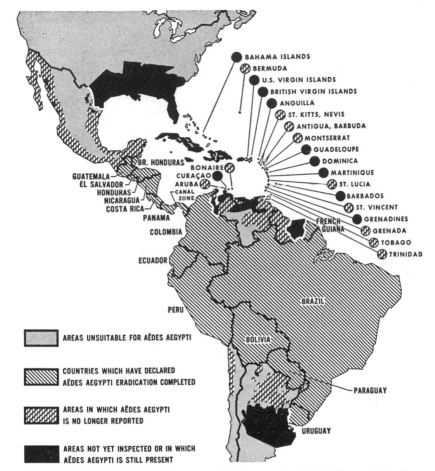

Figure 5. Status of the *Aedes aegypti* eradication campaign in the Western Hemisphere in December 1960. "*Aedes aegypti* eradication completed" signifies that eradication has been verified in accordance with the standards established by the Pan American Sanitary Bureau. (Pan American Health Organization) (1)

Basic Program Needs

All eradication programs have many needs in common. These include the need for political stability, for popular support, for adequate organization, for logistic and technical backing, and usually for an efficient quarantine system to prevent reinfection of the cleared area. Most important of all, the efforts must be pushed to the limit until the last parasite has been eliminated. The last 5 per cent is as important as the first 95 per cent. Anything less than 100 per cent is not eradication.

Political stability. Eradication programs are usually long-term, often requiring international co-operation. Obviously, nations work together better if they are at peace and friendly. Political upheaval and war usually disrupt such projects, and in countries like Tibet or the Congo, eradication programs are not likely to succeed. However, the recent collaboration of so many countries on issues such as malaria and smallpox has shown that much can be done even in a troubled world.

Popular support. Obviously, a program of eradication, with all its costs and inconvenience, will not be successful if it does not have popular support, even in a small country. On a world scale, this task of ensuring popular support might well daunt the most fervid supporter of the principle were it not for the United Nations. It is only through the United Nations that the two programs of smallpox and malaria control have been adopted by the majority of people, and even then it is clear that some of the nations involved have only a lukewarm interest in the project, while mainland China, biggest of all countries, with its 600 million people, is not even in the United Nations.

Great difficulty arises in areas where an infection of global or continental significance is of no particular public health importance locally. It is difficult to persuade a community to put up the funds and make the effort required for something that causes little local inconvenience. For example, a few countries joined in malaria eradication only after some hesitation; for them, malaria was simply not a public health problem, and there was no public pressure to organize expensive measures to benefit neighboring countries.

The costly and time-consuming efforts made to eradicate *Aedes aegypti* mosquitoes in urban areas have been substantially successful in South America (10), but as there is no yellow fever in the United States, there is no public pressure to get rid of *Aedes aegypti* mosquitoes there (Figure 5) *

Nonetheless, the United States has an international obligation to eradicate this species of mosquito, for its representatives supported and voted for the resolution in the first meeting of the Directing

* Application for funds for total eradication of *Aedes aegypti* from the United States have again in 1963 been turned down.

Council of the Pan American Sanitary Organization, a meeting in which it was resolved that *Aedes aegypti* mosquitoes must be eradicated from the Americas (11). As long as there are *Aedes aegypti* mosquitoes in North America, there will always be a likelihood that they will reinfect the areas in South America that have been cleared.

Syphilis might be eradicated from the United States by means of antibiotics and technical services already available, but it is unlikely that the public would accept an eradication program.

Technology. Eradication in any particular country may be impractical because the government lacks the funds or the personnel or the equipment or the organization. In certain nations of Africa, southeast Asia, and other parts of the tropics, the number of physicians and other trained personnel may be too small even for routine tasks, let alone the difficult and burdensome techniques of eradication. When the total national budget is inadequate, the proportion allotted for health purposes is usually small.

Equipment may be scarce, not to mention spare parts and repair technicians. Transport is frequently difficult because of a scarcity of vehicles and drivers and even of passable roads. For eradication, it is not enough to reach most places; one must reach all places. Usually 95 per cent are reasonably accessible, but the remaining 5 per cent are equally important.

The administrative organization of the national health department in the country undertaking eradication procedures must be strong enough to carry the load. Usually, in underdeveloped countries, the department is so small that one man does work that should be done by ten. Frequently major duties are left to clerks, since no one else is available. To expect these overworked people to take on responsibility for a large additional program is to be overoptimistic.

It might be expected that foreign aid would supply the needed technicians, administrators, equipment, and supplies. This it can do to a large extent, but there is a crucial service that can be performed only by the host nation itself. For example, the first stages of a program are usually easy enough, with teams of workers, imported or trained by foreign technicians, spraying the countryside with insecticides, giving injections or vaccinations, or handing out pills, and with everyone pleased as the disease in question recedes. But when the foreign teams depart, the task of finishing the job and of continuing surveillance falls to the host government. Then the government needs an efficient health service, with trained doctors who, in the course of their duties, will spot and report any recurrence of the disease. This program of surveillance has to be carried on for years in order that recurrences may be promptly discovered and stamped out in time. This task may be beyond the scope of any foreign aid, and all too often the national health department simply cannot carry it out. The final results over a ten-year period might well be especially disappointing if the program had started off well.

Reintroduction of a pathogen is an obvious danger where the operation is limited to a country or a continent, with infection remaining in regions outside. The usual method is to enforce quarantine measures, but the volume and nature of travel nowadays, especially by air, is making quarantine increasingly ineffective.

Biologic Factors in Eradication

On the basis of modern evolutionary theory it may be assumed that all human infections are derived from ancestral animal infections, since man himself was once a non-human animal. All human infections have related pathogens still existing in animal hosts, and the nature of these animal pathogens to a large extent decides whether or not an infection can be eradicated. Man belongs to the order Primates, and his relatives the apes, the monkeys, and other primates share with him parasites that have been handed down from one generation to another from their common primate ancestor. Earlier in this book it has been suggested that these parasites include the intestinal protozoa, pinworms, herpes virus, malaria parasites, and so on (Theory 2). In addition, there is a sharing of parasites among animals in intimate contact in the same ecology, as, for example, between man and his domestic animals. Sometimes this sharing is continued without change in the form of parasite, and a new form of zoonoses is established, while in other instances a newly parasitized species of host will convey the parasite within its own population and in time a new strain will be selected that is largely specific to that host. Elsewhere it has been suggested that this is the way in which the pox viruses evolved among the animals brought together into man's ecology when man settled down and domesticated animals (Theory 6).

Some of these relationships are close indeed; others are not so close, and some are fairly distant. When any eradication of an infection is contemplated, it is essential that the evolution of the agent be studied to determine the nature of these relationships and the effect they will have on the final result of the program. Related animal infections can be grouped as follows:

1. *Identical.* These infections are the zoonoses. From the point of view of eradication they can be subdivided into infections of wild animals and infections of domestic animals. If wild animals are involved (as in rabies, yellow fever, plague, rickettsial infections, or salmonella infections), then eradication will be difficult if not impossible. If only domestic animals are involved (as in *Mycobacterium bovis* infections, brucellosis, and glanders), then "regional" eradication is easy, for all that is necessary is to test the animals and kill the reactors, or else immunize the stock. However, research may show that most infections in domestic animals occur also in wild animals, and that world eradication may be impossible.

2. *Closely related.* In nature, closely related species sharing the same ecologies compete with one another, and this must happen with parasites also. Possibly the distribution of each species is to a certain extent dependent on this interspecific competition. A zoonosis like yellow fever is related to a wide range of other arbor viruses and almost certainly is affected by them. This is the explanation sometimes proposed for the absence of yellow fever in India, where the facilities for spreading have existed for at least 2,000 years. If yellow-fever virus were completely eradicated from Africa, it might well be that related, competing viruses would emerge prominently in that area.

Parasites similar to malaria parasites of man exist in apes and monkeys. The question as to whether they are identical is a matter of urgent research at the moment, but in any event there is no question but that man can be infected with these parasites (Chapter 9). Should the human malaria parasites be eradicated but not the vectors, then, after the eradication measures had been halted, man would be reinfected from the primates. If these have identical parasites or if they have not, over a period of decades human parasites might re-evolve from parasites of the primate reservoirs. In either case, human malaria would be likely to reappear.

As to treponemal infections, the various species are probably mere variants of one basic organism, as argued in a later chapter. Interspecific competition may partially determine whether a population contracts yaws or syphilis. Eradication of yaws will probably result in an increase in syphilis.

3. *Substantially different.* An infection such as smallpox is closely related to infections in other animals in man's immediate ecology—

animals such as mice, cows, horses, sheep, or chickens. It is possible that all of these infections derive from a radiation of a single organism that occurred at the time man first settled down and domesticated animals (Theory 6). These organisms are now so highly adapted to their hosts, and conditions have so changed from those under which they evolved, that the possibility that smallpox would re-evolve appears to be remote. The chances, therefore, of permanent eradication of the infection seem good.

4. *Very remote relationships.* Organisms like the leprosy bacillus have probably been symbiotes of man and his predecessors over many millions of years, are closely adapted to man, and have no close relations in other animals. Once eradicated, the chance of their re-evolving is extremely small.

It is becoming increasingly recognized that an organism that has radiated into many species is more capable biologically of surviving than one which has only a few species (12). A large organismal group is well equipped to withstand the adversities of changing environments and to adapt to new conditions as they arise. This strength arises from the variety of genetic mechanisms present in the radiation, in contrast to the limited range of mechanisms for organismal groups with only a few species. In general, wide radiations are found mainly in the locations of origin of the ancestral organism, and only single species or narrow radiations are found in areas where the organism has been newly introduced, for it takes considerable time for new species to appear. Eradication procedures will therefore be easier to complete and more successful, in long-term effects, when employed against species of parasite or insect vectors that have colonized the area in recent times than when employed against species that have been established there perhaps for millions of years.

The program to eradicate *Anopheles gambiae* in Brazil was a success, possibly because the mosquito was an introduced species (13), while a similar program against *A. labranchiae* in Sardinia was a failure in the sense that the mosquito species was not completely eliminated, because the anopheles in Sardinia were indigenous to the island and probably had been there many thousands or even millions of years (14). In addition to the mosquitoes which have become adapted to feeding on man within recent times, there was the original native stock, still feeding on wild animals. These mosquitoes of the original stock were not greatly affected by the eradication program and, presumably, form a reservoir from which fresh strains of domestic mosquitoes will evolve now that the program has terminated. Similarly, eradication of *Aedes aegypti* is proceeding very well in South America, where it probably is a newcomer of only some 400 years' standing, and where wild strains in the forest are as yet unknown. The story would be different should a similar program be attempted in East Africa, where wild strains are well established in the forest.

It is sometimes said that when an organism has been reduced to very small numbers it cannot survive and will die out spontaneously. This idea is of practical importance in eradication programs, for the last few sources of infection are difficult to reach. It is probably often true as applied to animals that are genetically diploid, but not necessarily so with microorganisms that are haploid. For example, the whooping cranes are probably doomed to extinction merely because there are only about 40 of them left alive. Deleterious or lethal mutations will occur occasionally in them; since most will be recessive, those that do not result in death will be stored away without expressing themselves. The close in-breeding that occurs in so small a population as 40 will result in these recessive deleterious mutations becoming demonstrated in the phenotype, so that the birds will become increasingly unfit to survive. They will be saved only if the environment changes substantially in their favor.

With haploid organisms, this is not the case, for any mutation is likely to be expressed immediately in the phenotype, and if the mutation is sufficiently deleterious, the individual organism will fail to survive. The future population of the haploid organism will consist only of the descendants of those without the mutation, so that small numbers do not necessarily indicate that the population is doomed to become extinct.

In a vector-borne infection, the pathogen will die out if the density of the vector is too low. This is a well-recognized phenomenon in malaria, yellow fever, plague, and filaria, and usually in control programs there are indices, such as the *aegypti* or the *cheopis* indices, of the permissible levels of vector densities for control of the infections. Should the numbers of these vectors be kept permanently below the threshold levels, then in time the pathogens will be eradicated. However, in any large country there may be small local pockets where high density levels of the vectors may persist, even though the general level for the area is low, and in an eradication program these must be sought for diligently. These pockets will not be so important in an infection like yellow fever, where the infectious process in the host is brief and the host population soon becomes immune to the pathogen, but they can be extremely important in malaria and filaria, where the host can carry the parasites for years.

Certain infections have been known to dwindle to small numbers and then disappear spontaneously. The extinction, however, was not due to the parasite population's falling below a hypothetical numerical threshold but to the parasites having lost their fitness to survive in the environment. "Fitness" can be defined as an organism's capacity to produce regularly as many viable members in one generation as in the preceding generation, for if it produces fewer in each succeeding generation, it will become extinct. Changes in environment and in behavior in places such as England and the United States in the past hundred years have tipped the balance against many parasites such as lice, the malaria parasite, the cholera vibrio, bubonic plague bacilli, and tubercle bacilli, and these infections, if they have not completely disappeared, are becoming less and less frequent. This process is clearly due to environmental changes and not to mere smallness in numbers of the parasites; the paucity of the organisms in the closing stages is merely the final step in a continuing process.

In a country where conditions favor the parasite, the elimination of this last trace of the infection can be extremely troublesome; yet until it has been accomplished, the campaign will not be a success. If the operating procedures are stopped prematurely, the infection will return, and either the program will have to be recommenced or else all the effort will have been wasted. In Ceylon, anti-mosquito measures were instituted in 1945 with the then newly available residual insecticide DDT, and the results exceeded expectations, for within one year there was a dramatic fall in the incidence of malaria. After a while the general spraying was stopped because of the increasing resistance of the mosquitoes, and reliance was placed on a surveillance system, with spraying of local infected areas. However, the malaria did not dwindle and vanish as expected but continued, and at the end of ten years it was still present in certain small foci (15). Malaria had been controlled but not eradicated. More vigorous measures are now being taken to discover and deal with these small foci.

The story has been much the same in Haiti, where yaws eradication is being attempted (Plate III). There had been 45,356 cases of yaws reported in 1949 on the island; in 1950 the general population had been given penicillin, and in 1953 only about 400 cases of yaws could be found. Every year since then the program has continued, and the early eradication of yaws has been eagerly expected, but each year up to 1959 there continued to be a hard core of about 300 cases. In nearby Jamaica, the yaws eradication program had made considerable progress when the teams for checking and surveillance were withdrawn prematurely. In 1959, 415 new cases of infectious yaws were reported, and the program had to be resumed (see Chapter 7).

Cincinnati was the first large city in the U.S. to try out the Sabin oral poliomyelitis vaccine. As an experiment, in 1960, about 200,000 children and young persons up to the age of 18 years were given the vaccine in a mass program. There had already been similar mass campaigns in 1955–56 for the Salk vaccine, and both then and in 1961 the public responded well to the intensive publicity programs. In 1960, a surveillance for cases of possible poliomyelitis was maintained by Dr. Albert L. Sabin and no case indigenous to Cincinnati was found. In 1961, it was necessary to immunize the infants born since the previous program, and again an intensive publicity campaign produced a satisfactory response as measured by the number of infants immunized. I continued the surveillance in 1961 on the same lines as had Sabin in the previous year and for the second year found no case of poliomyelitis indigenous to Cincinnati (see Chapter 9).

In 1962, it was a different story. By now the public had been exposed to the maximum publicity on polio for a series of years beginning in 1955 and had become apathetic on the subject. Furthermore, there had been no case in the city for two years and the general impression had arisen that there was no need for more immunization. The spring program in 1962 to immunize the infants and immigrants from outside the city was given the usual prominence in the press, radio, and on television, but the response was very poor, and obviously below what was needed on a long term basis for the continued elimination of the disease. It was not until the polio season started and a six-month-old baby that had not been immunized developed the disease—possibly outside of the city—that the citizens became alerted to the danger and the Academy of Medicine organized a mass campaign that immunized about two hundred thousand persons of all ages.

This kind of experience underlines the difficulties in the later stages of an eradication program. Once the first enthusiasm for the program has dwindled and the disease to a large extent has disappeared, it is difficult to keep the teams in the field and at a high level of efficiency. The mode of transmission may be difficult to see, so that cases pop up in unexpected places, and often supreme efforts are necessary to bring the transmitting agent to light. Soper has called this level of infectivity the "threshold of visibility" below which the mode of transmission of the infection cannot be seen with routine methods (13), and it is this that causes campaigns to drag on year after year when, according to all expectations, they should have been completed.

Eradication in Practice

Small islands are obviously the places where eradication efforts can best be made, for there the problems are clear-cut and quarantine measures are easiest to enforce. In England, several infections have been deliberately eliminated, including smallpox, rabies, and glanders, while typhus, plague, relapsing fever, malaria, cholera, and possibly leprosy have vanished, probably as a result of changing environments and habits. Smallpox was everywhere in England in the eighteenth century, but in 1853 vaccination was made compulsory. By 1871 the annual death rate per million people was down to 1,012, and in the ten-year period 1911–20, not a single death was reported. However, a very mild form was common during the 1920's (16). Vaccination is no longer compulsory and the immunity status of the nation is no longer so high, so that introduced infections every few years cause small outbreaks. The most recent one was started by Pakistani immigrants in 1961. However, smallpox still is not an endemic disease.

Glanders in England was eliminated by slaughtering all horses with the infection.

There has been almost no plague in England since the seventeenth century, partially as a result of the change in the species of rats in the island, and partially because of the vigorous campaigns at ports to keep out foreign rats. However, in the early 1900's, sylvatic plague was discovered in East Anglia, where a handful of human cases was diagnosed, and this persisted for a few years until it died out spontaneously. Presumably it had been introduced at a nearby port.

Higher standards of living and greater cleanliness were responsible for the disappearance of typhus and relapsing fever, for body-lice infestations are uncommon, although infestation with head lice still is found. Cholera has not been seen since the 1860's as a consequence of improvements in sewage disposal and management of water supply. Malaria has disappeared, partially because of the draining of the marshes and partially because its foothold in the country was always precarious as a result of the low summer temperatures. Also, the vector mosquitoes prefer feeding on animals to feeding on human beings.

Ceylon is another island with a good record of eradication of infections. Within the past 20 years, smallpox, plague, and cholera have all been wiped out, although each is likely to be reintroduced from time to time from India, which is only 18 miles away, across the Palk Strait. Smallpox was dealt with by maintaining high levels of vaccination immunity. Cholera and plague were both introduced infections which responded well to orthodox public health measures. The plague-carrying fleas had been imported from India and were limited to the port area of Colombo and to one or two small sites on the coast; rat-control measures have caused the infection to die out (17).

As for eradication on a regional scale, in America north of Mexico, several infections have disappeared. The last reported case of smallpox authenticated by isolation of the virus was in 1949 in Hidalgo County, Texas (18). Malaria dwindled with drainage of swamps and mosquito-proofing of homes. Control projects such as those of the Tennessee Valley Authority and the malaria control in war areas were also effective, so that by the end of World War II the surprising discovery was made that, without widespread use of DDT, malaria as an indigenous infection had practically ceased to exist, although it is continually being imported (19).

Yellow fever was easily eradicated in the United States, once the mosquito vector had been identified; the last cases of yellow fever were in New Orleans when about 1,000 deaths occurred (8).

There has been no cholera for a hundred years.

Quarantine

When a region, such as a country or continent, has rid itself successfully of some pathogen, the major question is whether or not it can resist reseeding of its population with that pathogen. The classic answer to the problem is that invented by the Venetians in which an entering traveler is kept isolated for 40 days or "quarantined." Unfortunately, modern methods of travel makes mockery of such old-fashioned techniques. Even the complex systems of inspection and immunization certificates used today by most immigration authorities at air and sea ports are proving increasingly inadequate. There is simply no practical rapid means of telling if a traveler is carrying organisms such as treponemes, malaria parasite, enteroviruses including poliovirus, hookworms, blood flukes, typhoid organisms, respiratory viruses, cholera vibrios, etc. Even in such a relatively simple matter as smallpox, the recent incident at New York Airport is instructive—a boy traveling from Brazil to Canada passed through the quarantine barrier carrying a smallpox certificate issued in Brazil, but nonetheless developed smallpox by the time he arrived in Canada. The boy had not, in fact, been vaccinated in Brazil, since the doctor who signed the certificate did not believe in it.

It is now possible to travel by jet plane from one continent to any of the others well within the incubation period of any of the major infections, and there is no means of detecting the incubating infection. With travel becoming increasingly popular, the task of keeping a country free of infections is growing that much more difficult. Of course the mere introduction of a pathogen into a country does not mean that it will spread there and establish itself. As mentioned elsewhere in this book, there are thousands of people in New York alone who are carrying parasites such as the blood fluke *Schistosoma* and the hookworm *Ankylostoma,* but these helminths cannot establish themselves in New York, since the means of transmission is lacking. Similarly, after World War II and the Korean War, many soldiers who had served overseas returned to the U.S. infected with malaria or filaria parasites, but the conditions for the establishment of these indigenous infections were adverse so that they just died out. But where conditions are favorable, as for smallpox, diphtheria, whooping cough, or polio, in a community that has abandoned the appropriate immunization measures, then it might take only one infected person to set off a disastrous epidemic. Yet until the immunizations are abandoned, eradication as defined here has not been attained. The main problem therefore in regional eradication is not so much finding a way to get rid of the infections in the first place, for the tools we have now are enough in most instances, but to discover means of identifying rapidly at the ports of entry which of the entering travelers are in an infectious state.

This matter was discussed at the first meeting of the Committee on Eradication of the American Public Health Association in Miami, October 1962. Dr. Fred L. Soper suggested that a more important matter than quarantine was the establishment of buffer zones around the free area. This had worked successfully in South America in the case of *Aedes aegypti:* once a place had been cleared of the mosquitoes, work was immediately begun on the areas on its borders. In this way the freed area was constantly being expanded and fewer and fewer mosquitoes found their way to the center. This is in fact what we are encouraging in Cincinnati in connection with our tuberculosis eradication which is described in a later chapter. The small townships within our borders or immediately adjoining them are being invited to participate in the program, both for their own benefit and to act as buffers between the city and the non-participating countryside around the city. Yet this can be only part of the answer, for people nowadays travel immense distances, as for example the boy with smallpox from Brazil. Such travelers skip over the buffer areas. And one of the reasons why South America has been able to make such progress in the *Aedes aegypti* campaigns is that reinfestation no longer occurs from Africa as it did in the old days. In the era of the sailing ship, water supplies were carried in barrels that were ideal for the breeding of *A. aegypti* and that was presumably how the mosquitoes crossed the South Atlantic in the first place. Today's ships have special water tanks that do not permit such breeding, so that a substantial ocean barrier prevents reinfestation of South America from Africa.

The answer to reinfection of regions cleared of infection lies in the invention of methods of rapid screening for these infections at ports of entry, the building up of cleared buffer areas as suggested by Dr. Soper, the rendering of environments to be unsuitable for infection as has happened for malaria in the U.S., or best of all, eradication on a world scale.

Conclusions

Eradication has been demonstrated many times to be entirely practical within certain limits, even with the techniques of today. Modern research is proceeding so quickly that many tasks that now seem impossible or extremely tedious and time-consuming may tomorrow be quite simple and quite rapidly performed. Most of the practical difficulties listed earlier in this article may be resolved in one or two decades.

Presumably, there will be rapid improvement in such areas as transport, logistics, and the strengthening of health services. Tasks such as the inoculation of people by the tens of millions will be speeded up by machines such as the hypospray jet injector. The dosing of people with drugs through additions to food or drink will make mass chemotherapy a practical matter. The development of live vaccines that can be given orally to babies soon after birth may immunize the populations of the world against many viruses. Such techniques, which are emerging in the laboratory today, may be available for use in the field in the near future.

Therefore, we can look forward with confidence to a considerable degree of freedom from infectious diseases at a time not too far in the future. Indeed, if the present pace of research and the present increase in the world's wealth continue, and if we suffer no major calamities such as an atomic war or an uncontrolled population explosion, then it seems reasonable to anticipate that within some measurable time, such as 100 years, all the major infections will have disappeared. This desirable goal will not be easily reached, for the difficulties are many, and unpleasant surprises are inevitable. Most of all there must be very much more research. And even as we are successfully eliminating one set of infections, new ones will almost certainly appear, for we live in a world swarming with potential pathogens in many forms. Evolution is not merely something that happened in the past; it is an essential part of both the present and the future, so that out of all the microorganisms that are continually seeking to invade our bodies, one that is favored by changing conditions will occasionally succeed. Always we will have to be on our guard, watching for signs of danger among the potential pathogens and stamping out the latest comer among them in the small focus in which it is evolving, and before it has the opportunity to spread across the world.

REFERENCES

1. COCKBURN, T. A.: Eradication of infectious diseases. Science, 1961, **133:** 1050–58.
2. SOPER, F. L.: Tuberculosis eradication. Amer. J. Public Health, 1962, **52:** 734–45.
3. W.H.O. Techn. Rep. Ser. No. **123,** 1957.
4. W.H.O. Techn. Rep. Ser. No. **162,** 1959.
5. W.H.O. Techn. Rep., 1960.
6. HAGAN, W. A.: The control and eradication of animal diseases in USA. Ann. Rev. Microbiol., 1958, **12:** 127–44.
7. VANE, W. F. M.: Statement in Parliament quoted in Brit. Med. J., June 2, 1962.
8. STRODE, G. K.: *Yellow Fever.* McGraw-Hill, New York, 1951.
9. SOPER, F. L. AND WILSON, D. B.: *Anopheles gambiae in Brazil 1930–1940.* Rockefeller Foundation, New York, 1943.
10. DIRECTOR, PAN AMERICAN SANITARY BUREAU: *Annual Report,* Washington, D.C., 1959.
11. Final reports of the first, second, and third meetings of the Directing Council, Pan American Sanitary Organization: Pan American Sanitary Bureau Publication No. 247. (1950), p. 3.

12. BATES, M.: in *Evolution after Darwin*, S. Tax, Ed., Univ. of Chicago Press, Chicago, 1960, p. 565.
13. SOPER, F. L.: The epidemiology of a disappearing disease: malaria. Amer. J. Trop. Med. & Hyg., 1960, **9:** 357–66.
14. LOGAN, J. A.: *The Sardinian Project.* The Johns Hopkins Press, Baltimore, 1953.
15. KARUNARATNE, W. A.: The influence of malaria control on vital statistics in Ceylon. J. Trop. Med. & Hyg., 1959, **62:** 79–85.
16. Report of the Committee on Vaccination, Ministry of Health. H.M. Stationery Office, London, 1928.
17. HIRST, L. F.: *The Conquest of Plague.* Clarendon, Oxford, 1953.
18. IRONS, J. V., SULLIVAN, T. D., COOK, E. B. M., COX, G. W. AND HALE, R. A.: Outbreak of smallpox in the Lower Rio Grande of Texas in 1949. Amer. J. Public Health, 1953, **43:** 25.
19. WILLIAMS, L. L.: Malaria eradication in the United States. Amer. J. Public Health, 1962, **53:** 17–21.

CHAPTER 7

The Treponematoses

THE PRINCIPLES GIVEN in the previous chapters will now be illustrated by applying them to a single group of infections, the treponematoses, beginning with the parasites as free-living organisms and following them through the ages to the present. The possibility of eradicating some or all of them will then be analyzed. Most of the theories listed in Chapters 4 and 5 will be employed. This description of the evolution of *Treponema* is based on the concept of a species described in Chapter 6.

The Treponematoses, as the name indicates, are a group of infections caused by organisms of the genus *Treponema*. There are several species of this genus listed in Bergey's *Manual of Determinative Bacteriology*, some being commensals, others mildly pathogenic for man, while three are associated with the principle diseases of the treponematoses: syphilis, yaws, and pinta. Recently a free-living form has been discovered. In many parts of the world there are variants of the non-venereal type of disease, and these are given varying names locally, such as bejel in Arabia, and irkinja in the Australia aborigine. In recent times, the idea has developed that many or all of these infections are in fact merely forms or variants of one basic infection, the differences being due chiefly to modes of transmission, climate, geography, humidity, etc. Traditionally, syphilis has been linked with the name of Columbus, whose men were supposed to have brought the infection back to Europe from the Americas.

The Remote Origin of the Treponematoses

It is regarded as axiomatic that all parasites are descended from free-living forms (Theory 1), so that it is in the soil or water that one must look for the original ancestor of the treponemes. It is unlikely that the free-living ancestors of *Treponema* still exist, but probable that some free-living descendants still survive with the same basic characteristics. This suggestion was made some years ago (1) and recently this has been confirmed by the discovery of such a free-living form of organism. Veldkamp had been studying organisms in mud and came across a new organism that seemed intermediate between *Borrelia* and *Treponema*. He described it as an anaerobic free-living Spirochaete of the genus *Treponema* and gave it the name *T. zuelzerae* (2).

The correctness of the placing of this organism in the genus *Treponema* has been confirmed by the finding that it possesses the Reiter antigen (3). The antigen of Reiter's treponeme (non-pathogenic, cultural strain) is the one described by D'Alessandro (4) as being group specific for both the pathogenic as well as the non-pathogenic cultural treponemes. Its possession by the free-living organism is therefore solid evidence for the claim that *T. zuelzerae* is indeed a treponeme of the same genus as the others.

The development of symbiosis between the free-living forms and the larger animals undoubtedly took place many millions of years ago, and probably the first sites to be occupied were the skin and orifices of the bodies of animals living in or ingesting the soil or water contaminated with the free-living forms. For a free-living form to jump at one stage to be a pathogen is probably a rare event, and the most likely possibility is that in the course of millions of years parasitic variants of the commensals slowly evolved in a number of different animals and orifices until there developed the families, genera, and species of the present-day order.

Once symbiosis has become established between a large animal and a microbe, there are two main ways in which the smaller partner can spread to new species of the animal. There can be direct horizontal spread to other animal species in the same ecology, or vertical spread throughout an adaptive radiation as the larger partner divides into new species over periods of millions of years as described in the chapter on paleoepidemiology. If man inherited his treponemes vertically from his remote primate ancestors, then a survey of the Order Primates would show that apes, monkeys, and other members were also hosts to species of *Treponema*. These would not necessarily be pathogens. If, however, he has been infected from some other animal in recent times, the other animal stock will have the related ancestral treponemes and the primate order would not generally be infected. Unfortunately, our knowledge of the distribution of treponemes throughout nature is extremely scanty, so that we cannot tell which of these two possibilities is correct. The rabbits have a treponeme closely related to that of man, but until further surveys have been made, we cannot tell whether man was parasitized from the rabbits or the rabbits from man, or both from some reservoir as yet unknown. As mentioned in Chapter 2, rabbits have been domesticated since Roman times.

Treponemes and the Genus Homo

It is generally accepted that before the days of Columbus there were treponemal infections both in the Old World (which included Africa and Asia) and in the New World of the Americas. No one can doubt that pinta has been in Central America for a very long time, while ancient bones with some form of treponemal pathology have been uncovered in various parts of the Old World. Since the organisms responsible for the diseases must have descended from a common ancestor, as tacitly assumed by placing the treponemal species in one genus, there must have been some connection between the infections; the difficulty is in finding some link between the populations on the two great land masses. It is possible to imagine that some recent group of migrants—such as the Eskimos, or the Vikings who crossed the North Atlantic to Greenland, or some hypothetical travelers of the Pacific—were responsible for introducing the treponemes to the New World, but there is no evidence to support such an idea. The only other likelihood is that the original settlers of the New World were already infected when they first crossed the Bering land bridge tens of thousands of years ago.

As described in Chapter 2, modern man is thought to have appeared about 100,000 years ago, either in Africa or Asia, and to have traveled over the world at a time when the sea level was much lower than it is now. He would take many of his parasites with him and among them probably would be some form of treponeme. In other words, treponemes were not carried by Columbus or any one else in recent times from one continent to infect another for the first time; they were already in every place reached by man before the era of ocean travel. There is no other acceptable way of explaining the distribution of pinta in America and yaws in much of the rest of the world before this era of travel and discovery opened. This being the most likely possibility, the main task remaining is to explain how the ancestral organism of the earliest stock of modern man came to produce such differing diseases in various parts of the world.

Elsewhere, it has been proposed that a host exposed to a parasite becomes genetically resistant to that parasite, the resistance being handed down from one generation to another and increasing or decreasing according to the amount of handicap given it by the parasite in the struggle for existence. If the host is severely handicapped, the genetic resistance might reach considerable proportions in only a few generations. From these generalities it can be concluded that, after a few thousand years of isolation from one another, the various human races would differ in their reactions to the treponemes infecting them. Similarly the pathogens would also produce differences, so that the disease picture could be expected to differ from one isolate to another.

The group of people geographically isolated for the longest period were those in America, for even when the Bering land bridge was still open, the number of individuals traveling by it must always have been small. The addition of such small quantities of new human genetic variants to the general mass of those already in Central America could have had little effect for some thousands of years before the land bridge was broken. It is suggested that pinta is the result of this process of geographical isolation, and the reason for its existing in so limited an area as Central America is that not only does the organism differ from those in other parts of the world, but so also does the human host and his reaction to his parasite.

This concept is supported by two facts: first, that the pinta organism varies from all other treponemes by a greater degree than others do, being the only one that has so far resisted all efforts to adapt it to a laboratory animal; and secondly, that pinta is still confined largely to its original home in Central America in spite of ample opportunity for it to spread in modern times. Pinta-like lesions are found in treponemal disease all over the world, but the full picture of the disease spread through a population is found only in Central America, and no other satisfactory explanation for this is forthcoming except that the full disease is produced only when the proper human host is infected. Such a host is found only in Central America.

Geographical isolation as a cause of speciation in parasites of the human races is of course not confined to the treponemes. A good example of the same process occuring at the same time as the variations in the treponemes is found in the body lice. Studies have shown that the lice vary from one human race to another, with those of the white races of the Eurasian land mass differing from those of all other races. The ones of the American Indian are distinctive and most closely resemble those of the yellow races. The African lice differ most of all, being black and only half the size of those of the white races (5).

Ecological separation as distinct from geographical separation is well demonstrated by the incidence of yaws and venereal syphilis in the temperate regions. There is no geographical barrier separating these two infections. In certain locations in the syphilis sectors, a non-venereal yaws-like treponemal infection exists in populations where the hygiene is bad; in endemic yaws regions, groups with high standards of living, such as Europeans, rarely have yaws but can acquire venereal syphilis. Some hundreds of years ago, non-venereal syphilis, usually called "sibbens," was not uncommon in the remoter parts of Great Britain (6).

The explanation given here is that, since the treponeme is a very delicate organism that cannot exist for long periods away from its human host, it must have almost direct routes of transmission from body to body, and the wearing of clothes must interfere drastically with this process and cut down the survival potential of the organisms. In warm climates where clothes are not worn, skin to skin transmission is obviously practical, but it is suggested that where clothes are worn, in such places as the temperate climates or among wealthier classes (such as the European) in the tropics, the yaws type of organism cannot survive. Exceptions to this would be in communities where overcrowding is intense and many people sleep together, as they did in the old days in Great Britain, or where special customs and rites provide for almost direct transmission, as in the "custom syphilis" in Russia and the Balkans.

If a yaws treponeme were imported to Europe, as indeed must happen frequently in these days of air and sea travel, it would find itself at a biological disadvantage and would soon die out. The syphilis organism in highly endemic yaws areas, such as West Africa, will find only a limited cultural group of persons for its permanent survival, for as soon as it is taken to peoples in which yaws is highly endemic, it will either itself become transmissible by non-venereal means, or soon die out, since most of the population will have become immune to yaws before puberty. Intermediate zones would occur where the conditions were not fully favorable to either infection and both would exist side by side.

Australia was also isolated, but not to the same extent as America. The inhabitants of that continent almost certainly arrived there by boat, island-hopping over the original narrow channel, and the process must have continued as the channel grew wider. The Polynesians arrived on the scene with ocean-going craft in that general area about one and a half thousand years ago and undoubtedly visited Australia. How far the irkinja of Australia is due to isolation and how much it has been affected by later importations, it is difficult to say.

The treponemal infections of man in the very early days would differ from those of the present time, because the populations were so much smaller. One of the theories expressed earlier (Theory 4) is that the nature of an infection is influenced by the size of the population, being chronic in small populations and acute in large ones. In migrant groups of small size dependent on hunting for food, only infections of a saprophytic nature or low-grade pathogenicity could survive, but as agriculture and the domestication of animals were discovered, the populations increased and more acute strains of pathogens could exist. Even then, it must be remembered that the total population of both Americas at the time of Columbus did not exceed about eight million people (7, 8), and that the fastest rate of travel was that of a man's legs, for there were no horses. Under these conditions, only chronic infections like pinta or low-grade sores could survive. Yaws is a relatively acute infection, probably because it had a huge population to support it. At the time of Columbus there were possibly as many people in West Africa alone as in the whole of the Americas.

The Infections in Modern Times

By about A.D. 1000, the position was probably as follows. Treponemes would exist either as commensals or parasites on all continents of the world, but because of the smallness of the populations in most parts, any disease would be of a mild type and chronic in nature. As the numbers of people in the Old World rose, more acute infections would be selected, and because of the unhygienic conditions prevailing these would be spread by direct personal contact at an early age. The squalor in both the towns and the countrysides of those days was considerable, and in areas exposed to warfare the people crowded into fortified towns under conditions of overcrowding that were appalling. This continued until the discovery of gunpowder made city walls no longer a refuge from attack, so that towns expanded beyond their previous confines and overcrowding diminished, until the Crusades opened the eyes of Europeans to higher standards of personal comfort, and until the Renaissance and the Reformation opened men's minds to new ways of thinking and living. By 1492, unhygienic environments still prevailed, but living conditions had made a big advance on what had gone before, and this must have affected the transmission of treponemes.

Prior to that time, nudity had not been a matter for shame among the Germanic (9) and British peoples (10), so it was normal for peoples of both sexes to gather in communal bathhouses and share the same baths. Without thinking it in any way unusual, a whole family —father, mother, sons, and daughters, would walk unclothed down the street from the home to the bathhouse. At night, the whole family group would sleep in one room with several sharing a bed and all sleeping naked. Nor would this be limited to the family, but also the servants, friends, guests, and even passing travelers would also be there. Detailed rules of etiquette existed on how to behave when sharing a bed with a stranger. For example, the person with the highest rank would be offered the place at the edge of the bed. Special night clothes were not worn, and it was thought odd if a person slept in the same shirt that he wore in the day (10). Even in the great family households, there was little privacy; the lower servants slept in the great hall or in any outhouse they could find open, while those of higher rank used a common dormitory. In the household of the great Earls of Northumberland as late as the middle of the sixteenth century, the regulations required the chaplains to sleep two, and the choir boys three, to a bed (11). Such conditions were ideal for the spread of infections requiring intimate contact for person-to-person spread, and treponemes would have no difficulty in surviving by non-venereal transmissions. As late as the middle of the seventeenth century, this form of life still persisted in remote parts of the British Isles, and in such areas a yaws-like disease called "sibbens" after its raspberry appearance was not uncommon. For example, it was recorded that Oliver Cromwell's troops became infected with this disease when occupying such remote areas (6).

The great change may have been largely due to religious influences, for the new Protestant movement attacked the immorality that was to be found in the communal bathhouses and common sleeping rooms, and the Catholic Church soon followed suit. Under the attacks of the clergy, nudity in public became a matter for shame and the bathhouses largely ceased to be communal affairs. For the first time, people began wearing night dresses as a routine and requiring privacy during the sleeping hours. Even in inns where of necessity travelers had to share beds with any fellow travelers, people began expecting better conditions, so that by the middle of the eighteenth century one writer remarked that it was unusual to have to share a bed in an inn (9).

Such changes could well affect the passage of treponemes from one person to another, and it is suggested here that, in the changing circumstances, those treponemes in the temperate zones that depended on direct skin-to-skin transmission were at a biological disadvantage and largely died out. Those that would survive would be the hardier saprophytes and a strain that had developed venereal transmission. Such a venereal strain would have always been a potential possibility, for yaws lesions not uncommonly occur on the penis or female sex organs so that the chances of venereally transmitted yaws lesions are quite considerable. A distinctive strain would not emerge as an entity so long as it was not isolated from the other treponemes, for it would interbreed with them and lose its identity. Once the others were out of the way, syphilis in its modern form would appear. In this concept, the relationship of the discovery of America and the first appearance of syphilis would not be that of cause and effect, but both would be consequences of one common factor, the change in knowledge, ideas, and culture resulting from the Renaissance and the Reformation. The relationship with the voyage of Columbus would be no coincidence, since it too was a product of the Renaissance.

Syphilis differs from yaws and pinta in certain significant respects; congenital infection of the fetus occurs, and also lesions of the internal organs such as the central nervous system, aorta, bones, and indeed any part of the body. The reasons for these are not known and indeed it is a perplexing problem, for from the point of view of survival of the organism, such infections are of no obvious importance. The chances are infinitely small of an individual treponeme in a gumma of the liver or brain ever reaching the outside world and finding a new host to infect.

So far as the congenital infections of syphilis are concerned, it is not too difficult to imagine a possible sequence of events. Basically, the syphilis treponeme exists by transmission during sex contact, and if any particular strain regularly fails to infect the appropriate section of mucous membrance in the sex organs, it will become extinct. The mere fact that venereal syphilis exists as a distinct and separate entity (with only the occasional extragenital transmission) indicates that a genitotropic strain of treponeme has evolved under the influence of natural selection. The diagnosis of syphilis in a person indicates that the treponemes in that person have been passed down by venereal transmission (with only a rare exception) through 20 or 50 generations. In women, this means that in all established strains, the treponeme must have access to the mucous membrane of the vagina. This could be achieved either by a solitary sore in the vagina or by infection of the uterus. To the treponeme, infection of the uterus has a strong survival value since it ensures a constant stream of organisms to the vagina, where transmission takes place. In other words, in syphilis a strain of treponeme has evolved through natural selection whose main characteristic is that it infects the sex organs; all those that do not do this become extinct. It follows as a natural result that the fetus inside the infected uterus would also be invaded.

It is suggested here that the invasion of the internal organs so characteristic of syphilis is a result of this congenital infection, by development of organotropic strains through passage of the trepo-nemes through series of fetuses. The possibility of producing or-ganotropic strains through passage through fetuses does not seem too remote when it is remembered that a hundred years ago it was almost normal for one woman to have a dozen pregnancies, and not uncommon to have two dozen. But before proceeding farther, the background for this idea has to be explored.

The early embryo is embedded in its mother's tissues, and after about the third month the fetus is separated from its mother only by some delicate placental membranes that are obviously easily pene-trated by the treponeme. The exchange of treponemes between mother and fetus will not be merely a one-way process, so that the mother will also be infected from the fetus and the treponemes inside the mother will mate with those from the fetus and be altered by them. In a heavily infected fetus, every drop of blood coming along the umbilical cord to the placenta must be swarming with fetal trep-onemes. The environment in which the treponemes live in the fetus is considerably different from that in the mother; first, for much of the time there are for practical purposes no sex organs for the trep-onemes to infect; secondly, infection of the skin or mucous mem-brane of the fetus has little survival value for treponemes, for the organisms on the exterior of the fetus are at a disadvantage in that they may be cast off into the amniotic fluid with no way to the out-side world, while those that colonize the internal organs such as the liver and bones will have easy access back to the mother, along the wide open road of the umbilical cord.

These factors would influence the selection of mutants inside the fetus and produce a variant considerably different from that in the adult. The emphasis would be on treponemes adapted to the internal organs other than the sex organs and skin, and such a process continued, say, a dozen times in the lifetime of one woman would be quite enough to explain the characteristic internal lesions of syphilis. In yaws the process would occur occasionally as part of the general infection, so that the internal organs would be involved to some lesser extent.

Eradication

Eradication programs for various diseases of the treponematoses have been declared in several countries. Included in these are programs against yaws in Indonesia, Nigeria, and several islands in the West Indies, against pinta in Central America, and syphilis in the United States. A World Forum on Syphilis and the Treponematoses was held in Washington, D.C., in September 1962, although the accent was on syphilis since most of the speakers came from the United States.

The eradication of syphilis apparently is now the aim of the U.S. Public Health Service, so far as the continental United States is concerned. Such a policy was a recommendation of the Task Force on Syphilis under the chairmanship of Dr. Leona Baumgartner and appointed by the Surgeon General of the U.S. Public Health Service. Eradication was the main theme of the World Forum on Treponematoses held in September 1962 in Washington, D.C. In spite of this, there has been no general agreement as to what is meant precisely by "eradication." It is, therefore, thought proper at this time to discuss this matter of the concept of eradication as applied to syphilis, to review the varying interpretations given to the concept by different workers, and to ask, in fact, what is it that we are trying to do or should be trying to do. Badly needed at present is some clear statement on long range aims.

The debate over the word eradication is not one of semantics nor of mere academic interest, but rather one that can be measured in dollars and cents. If the word is taken to mean the pushing down of the disease to a very low level and keeping it at that level, then the operation must be regarded as a continuing one with substantial recurring costs. This is really an advanced stage of "control." If it means the complete wiping out of the pathogen in question under such conditions that all control measures can be abandoned, apart from a certain degree of surveillance, then the initial cost may be high while completing the program, but once it is achieved there are no recurring costs for the future.

Definition of Eradication

The Surgeon General of the U.S. Public Health Service in his directive to the Task Force used the phrase "eradication of syphilis as a public health problem" (12). This phrase implies that when the status of eradication has been achieved there will still be cases of syphilis remaining in the country. This in turn means that the expensive program of syphilis control will be continued indefinitely into the future. The present federal expenditure is about eight million dollars a year, and state, county, and city expenses must be added to this, making a substantial annual bill.

Dr. William J. Brown, in his opening address at the World Forum, defined eradication as the elimination of the last case of syphilis in the United States. This is obviously a much more ambitious target than that of the Surgeon General. Unfortunately, he did not discuss what would happen after the last case of syphilis had been eliminated from the country. The main problem of all local eradication programs is the prevention of reintroduction of fresh infections outside the eradication area. Dr. Brown did not mention how the reintroduction of syphilis in the United States from other parts of the world would be prevented, once the last case of syphilis had been discovered and treated. Presumably the whole anti-syphilis program by federal government, city, and other authorities would have to continue indefinitely to make certain that any recurrence of the disease would be quickly identified and dealt with.

In October 1961, the American Public Health Association held a seminar on the "Concept of Eradication" at their annual meeting in Detroit. A concept advanced by Dr. Alexander D. Langmuir and Dr. Justin Andrews reads as follows: "To achieve and maintain the eradication status of a specific disease within an area, it is necessary 1) to obstruct transmission until endemicity ceases, and 2) to prevent or nullify the re-establishment of the disease from carriers, relapsing cases, or imported sources of infection" (13). This statement goes further than that of Dr. Brown, in that it attempts to deal with the situation that arises when the last case of disease in question has been eliminated. It is to be noted, however, that here again there is implied the continuance of active measures for an indefinite period of time.

To illustrate the problem, let us compare the two infections of malaria and smallpox. Malaria was once a common disease in the United States and a considerable organization was created to control it. At the end of World War II, it was discovered, to everyone's surprise, that it had in fact disappeared from the country, so that active transmission within the U.S. border no longer occurred. Since then, all malaria control measures have been disbanded except for a certain degree of surveillance. This has proved practical, even though thousands of people infected with malaria parasites arrive in the United States every year. Smallpox likewise has disappeared from the United States. There has been no indigenous case proven by virus isolations for more than a decade. By the definition of Dr. Langmuir and Dr. Andrews, smallpox would have been eradicated: nevertheless, it is still necessary every year to vaccinate between five and ten million people in the United States at a great cost of money, a substantial amount of sickness from the vaccine, and even deaths each year.

TABLE 8. CINCINNATI HEALTH DEPARTMENT, V.D. QUESTIONNAIRE, OCTOBER, 1962

	Physicians replying		
	Number replying	Number in county	% Replying
Derm.	19	25	76.0
G.P.	204	262	77.5
Surg.	52	94	55.3
Int. Med.	142	237	59.9
Ob/Gyn.	52	60	86.7
Other Spec.	265	431	61.5
Osteopaths	19	26	73.1
Total	753	1,135	66.3

My own definition of eradication has been spelled out in some detail earlier. To me a disease is eradicated when all transmission of the infection from person to person has ceased under such conditions that no further efforts at control are required beyond a certain amount of surveillance. The infection has gone and does not return, even though no active measures are maintained. To me, malaria has been eradicated; smallpox has not been eradicated, since the immunization has to continue.

None of the concepts offered by various authorities as listed above can be considered as proper eradication so long as the active measures against syphilis have to be continued. They are merely advanced forms of control.

A joint statement in "Today's VD Control Problem" has been issued in 1963 by The Association of State and Territorial Health Officers, The American Venereal Disease Association, and The American Social Health Association. It is to be noted that throughout this statement the word "control" is used and the word "eradication" is scarcely mentioned.

Syphilis Today

In the Task Force report, the figure given for cases of primary and secondary syphilis for 1960 was 16,144. At the present moment a national survey has just been made by means of addressing questionnaires to all physicians in the United States asking details as to the number of cases seen by them.

In the meantime our Department in Cincinnati has already made such a survey and has gathered figures which show the reported cases in our area to be only a small fraction of the total diagnosed by physicians (14). Our Health Department questionnaire was sent to every physician in Hamilton County, in which the city of Cincinnati is located, and the conclusion reached was that in this one county alone, with a population of 864,121 in 1960, there were about 124 cases of primary or secondary syphilis diagnosed in the first nine months of 1962. The questionnaire merely asked how many new cases of venereal disease by type and stage had been seen by the physician in the first nine months of 1962, together with the physician's type of practice. The physician replying was not required to sign the reply nor give his name. It should be noted that of the 1,135 physicians in the county, 66.3 per cent of all of these replied (Table 8). The questionnaire showed that these physicians in private practice reported only one case in 12 of infectious syphilis seen by them (Table 9). This proportion held also for gonorrhea, but 40 per cent of tertiary syphilis was notified. Most of the cases reported to the Health Department came from the city's public clinics (Table 10). It was estimated that had 100 per cent of the physicians replied and had the survey covered twelve months of 1962 instead of nine months, then the total number of early syphilis cases diagnosed in Hamilton County would have been about 168, giving a rate of 20.8 per 100,000 population (assuming the incidence for the last three months of the year to be the same as that of the first nine months and that the physicians who did not reply diagnosed as many cases as those who did). This rate should be compared with 2.9 cases per 100,000 population for Ohio as was given in "Today's VD Control Problem."

TABLE 9. SYPHILIS—PRIMARY AND SECONDARY

Specialties	Number of cases previously rptd.	Number of cases rptd. in survey	% Column 1 column 2
Derm.	1	7	14.3%
G.P.	2	52	3.8%
Surg.	1	0	—
Int. Med.	1	9	11.1%
Ob/Gyn.	0	3	0.0%
Other Spec.	1	5	20.0%
Osteopaths	0	4	0.0%
Total	6	80	7.5%

This data from Hamilton County, Ohio, can be compared usefully with that resulting from a national survey completed in 1963 by the American Social Health Association. The results are fundamentally the same, although the national one was more restricted, being limited to members of the American Medical Association, the National Medical Association, and the American Osteopathic Associa-

TABLE 10. CASES OF VENEREAL DISEASE REPORTED TO CINCINNATI HEALTH DEPARTMENT JANUARY–SEPTEMBER 1962

	City clinics	Private physicians	Total
Syphilis Primary and secondary	16	6	22
Other	257	127	384
Gonorrhea	961	133	1,094

tion, while ours in Cincinnati covered all licensed practitioners in Hamilton County. The national survey questionnaire was sent to 172,000 doctors and 11,000 osteopaths and a 71.7 per cent response was obtained. Replies were received from 131,245 physicians, reporting (among other data) 13,930 cases of primary and secondary syphilis; only 1,576 have been notified, a percentage of 11.3. In Ohio, only

5.6 per cent of cases had been notified, as compared with the 7.5 per cent as found in our survey.

Much of the difficulty is with regard to notification on the point of confidentiality between the physician and patient. Some states have laws dealing with the confidentiality of records such as those dealing with V.D. Ohio is not one of these states. The fact is that under Ohio law none of the City Health Departments are privileged. Recently, I personally have received a subpoena to produce in court the findings of a patient alleged to have been in our V.D. Clinic. Until the Ohio law is amended with regard to confidentiality, physicians will be very reluctant to report cases to our department.

TABLE 11. SYPHILIS IN CALIFORNIA 1962 REPORTED BEFORE AND AFTER
LABORATORY NOTIFICATION REGULATION
(By Selected Local Health Jurisdictions.)

Project personnel assistance to jurisdictions	Primary and secondary syphilis		% Increase following regulation	Population July 1, 1962
	Before	After		
Total jurisdictions	819	1,065	30%	17,094,000
Jurisdictions with assistance	623	844	35%	8,894,100
Jurisdictions without assistance	196	221	12.8%	8,199,900

Section 2505, Title 17, California Administrative Code became effective April 25, 1962. It is assumed that the regulation did not become effectively implemented until some time after this date. For this reason (and because of the nature of the venereal disease reporting system) the pivotal date for this before-after comparison is arbitrarily established at June 30, 1962. Morbidity "before" the regulation is that reported during the six-month period January to June 1962; morbidity "after" the regulation is that reported during the six-month period July to December 1962.

Source: Preliminary data, VD Section, Bureau of Communicable Diseases, California Department of Public Health.
State of California, Department of Finance, Financial and Population Research Section, population estimates.

A great point was made by the Task Force of the compulsory reporting of all positive serologies by laboratories testing sera. For the past two years, the Cincinnati Health Department has been studying the situation with regards to such a regulation for the city area. There has been considerable opposition to the proposal. I have been told personally by physicians in various parts of the United States that if such a law is passed, they would send their sera to laboratories elsewhere. If the law were made applicable to the whole United States, they would send their sera to Canada or Mexico. They justify their position by stating that it is in the best interest of their patient to do so. They do not wish their patients to be harassed nor run the risk of having the nature of their illness disclosed to other persons.

If positive serologies were made reportable by law in Ohio, undoubtedly extra cases would be discovered which otherwise would go unreported. This is supported by the experience of the State of California, where the appropriate law became effective April 5, 1962 (see Table 11), and cases of primary and secondary syphilis reported increased by 30 per cent. Yet almost inevitably, the end result would be a "Black Market" in testing of possible syphilitic sera.

The fact is that any law is useless unless it will be either obeyed or enforced. The physicians of the United States obviously are not obeying the law requiring them to report syphilis, and there are no practical means available to make them obey the law. It must be very rare for any physician to be taken to court and punished for failing to report a case of syphilis. Certainly none of the authorities in our part of the Midwest would dream of doing such a thing. Even in Cincinnati we would not dare to push this matter to this logical conclusion, since the accused physician would claim, in perfect honesty, that he was acting in the best interest of his patient and his colleagues would probably support him. The whole medical profession in this area would be antagonized, and the net result of any such action would be a solid hostility which would have a markedly adverse effect on our other public health programs.

It would not be possible to enforce a law on reporting of positive sera unless inspectors were available to go around and study the records of the various laboratories. Even if we had the necessary staff to carry out this inspection, ways and means would be found to hide the data. It is not only likely that a "Black Market" in serologies would develop; in my opinion, this already probably exists in parts of the country. This is clearly shown by the results of the national survey. When the figures are broken down by states, it is quite obvious that reporting in those with laws about positive serologies is little better than those without such laws (Table 12).

The Reimportation of Infection from Abroad

Every day tens of thousands of people cross the borders of the United States. Substantial numbers of these people must have syphilis. There are no means available at the present moment to screen out these infected individuals and treat them before they have the opportunity of spreading their infection. Any talk of any form of eradication is useless until this problem of reimportation is solved.

There is no scientific or technical difficulty preventing reinfection of the country. All persons coming into the country could be given injections of antibiotics or their sera could be tested by some rapid screening method. The difficulty is that in this world of fast jet travel and difficult international relations, such means are simply not practical. At a crowded international airport, full of travelers from all

TABLE 12.* STATES WITH LAWS REQUIRING REPORTING OF POSITIVE SEROLOGIES. NUMBER OF CASES TREATED BY PHYSICIANS COMPARED WITH NUMBER REPORTED 1962, PRIMARY AND SECONDARY SYPHILIS ONLY

	No. of physicians replying in survey who diagnosed syphilis	No. of cases treated	No. reported	% reported
Total U.S.A.	7,082	13,930	1,576	11.3
California	817	1,567	128	8.1
Connecticut	79	103	4	3.9
Illinois	291	515	88	17.1
Kentucky	70	105	7	6.7
Maine	30	55	3	5.4
Michigan	243	464	16	3.4
New York	1,013	1,807	389	21.5
North Carolina	178	358	60	16.8
Pennsylvania	479	937	52	5.5
South Carolina	97	226	56	24.8
Vermont	6	9	0	—
Virginia	156	293	23	7.8
Wisconsin	66	145	11	7.6
TOTALS FOR 13 STATES	3,525	6,584	837	12.7

* Data from Summary Report of a National Study of VD Incidence by the American Social Health Association.

countries, some of them on diplomatic visas, all kinds of non-scientific difficulties would arise. Yet until this problem has been solved, it is not justifiable to use the word eradication except as a hope for the future.

The big shock in the past decade has been the discovery of the considerable amount of syphilis being spread among homosexuals. The majority of the cases found in our city is now of this type, and apparently this is a national experience, judging by the remarks at the World Forum. The feeling there was that this was nothing new, but only that homosexuality was now becoming more "accepted" by society so that there is more inclination to report the disease than in the past. Table 13 is an example of what is being found in Cincinnati by our Venereal Disease investigators (15). It could be paralleled by similar studies in any other city in the U.S.

At the turn of the last century, homosexuality was a matter that

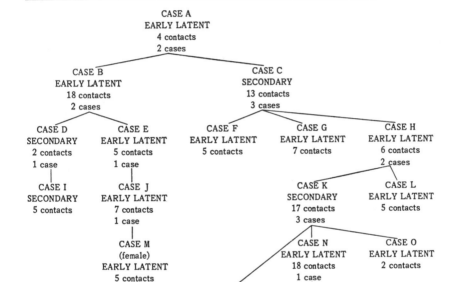

Table 13. An Early Syphilis Epidemiologic Chain Among Homosexual Males, Cincinnati 1962

simply was not discussed or spoken about. The trial of Oscar Wilde and his sentence of two years in Reading Jail was typical of the general attitude of the public in England and the Western world in general. Under such conditions it would have been almost impossible to have tracked down the spread of the infection in the manner shown in Table I. The position is so altered that now many homosexuals live openly together in a fashion that is relatively permanent and resembles normal childless marriage. Table 12 gives the impression of considerable promiscuity, but in fact, there seem to be many that are "true" to one another. Under the changed conditions, the improved reporting of diseases may well account for what at first sight seems to be a marked increase in the disease.

What are we trying to do with regard to syphilis? There is no question but that syphilis is a serious and increasing problem. Obviously, much money will have to be appropriated at all levels of government, and many trained personnel will have to be employed. Physicians must collaborate by reporting both diagnosed cases and positive serologies. New laws will have to be drawn up, passed by state legislatures, and enforced by local authorities. All this is very necessary. Having agreed to this, it is logical to ask what we hope to achieve by all this effort and how long must it be continued? In "Today's VD Control Problem," the following statement is made: "If the program can be further improved by providing increased personnel and other facilities, service and materials needed, the trend should be reversed and the curve of incidence started downward. This will happen, however, only if federal, state and city appropriations are increased to the level needed and maintained at that level for the period of years required to virtually eradicate the disease." There can be no quarrel with the intent of the statement, but one can wish that the time factor "period of years" had been stated more precisely, and that criteria had been provided to indicate the point at which "virtual" eradication would be reached.

In my opinion the following conclusions seem inevitable:

1. There is far more syphilis in this country than has been previously thought likely. The problem is, therefore, much more serious than it appeared before the national survey.

2. A much sharper concept of eradication is required. The target at which we should aim should be clearly defined. Vague terms such as "to virtually eradicate" or to "eradicate as a public health problem" should be discarded.

3. Syphilis eradication in the strict sense is not practical at present, according to my definition. Most likely syphilis will exist in the U.S. for several decades in the future. Any planning or appropriation of money should be made with this realization in mind.

4. Steps for making the reporting of positive serologies compulsory will almost certainly reveal a number of cases which now go unreported. However, the end result will probably be a

"black market" in sera testing, which in the long run will cause considerable trouble.

5. The laws in most states are inadequate to deal with the problem of syphilis. Perhaps the most important one deals with the confidentiality of reports. Until such legislation is enacted, physicians in Ohio and many other states in the Midwest will be extremely reluctant to disclose the names of their infected patients.

6. The eradication will not be possible until adequate steps have been taken to prevent the importation of infections from abroad.

7. The complete change in public attitude toward sex and venereal disease will be necessary before syphilis can be eradicated. Only when the disease is regarded as is polio or tuberculosis will the last case be discovered and treated.

Conclusion

There is more syphilis than is generally supposed.

The anti-syphilitic campaign will be a long one, measured in decades and not years. Accordingly, measures for dealing with the infection should be planned accordingly.

Overoptimism should be avoided.

Research is needed into the problem of introduction of the infection from abroad.

A primary task is the overhaul of state legislation, especially with regard to confidentiality of records.

Yaws

There is confused thinking on the status of the treponematoses. Most people seem to give lip service to the idea that all the varying kinds of treponematoses, yaws, syphilis, pinta, bejel and non-venereal syphilis, etc., are really all basically variants of one infection; in four days of continuous talking, I found no one at the World Forum who was ready to follow this to the logical conclusion in the practical application in the field. If yaws and syphilis are really closely related, and both exist in the same country and people, then efforts to eradicate one without touching the other are unrealistic. Suppose all the yaws treponemes are indeed successfully wiped out and the programs are abandoned either because the goal has been reached or because funds are no longer appropriated for the purpose, what will happen next?

Presumably the social conditions have not changed to any great extent, and the opportunities still exist for direct skin-to-skin transmission that permitted the yaws treponeme to flourish. Almost certainly the infection will either be reintroduced from neighboring areas that have not been cleared or else non-venereal transmission of syphilis will in time produce a form of disease that will be more or less indistinguishable from the original yaws.

The difficulties are well illustrated by the yaws eradication programs in the West Indies, as mentioned earlier in the chapter on the basic principles of eradication. In Haiti, the islanders were given injections of penicillin, and the cases of the disease dropped dramatically from 45,356 in 1949 to only about 400 in 1953. The final proclamation that eradication had been achieved was eagerly anticipated. In 1954, the Director of the Pan American Sanitary Bureau, in his Annual Report, could say "the eradication of yaws in Haiti is nearer than ever to a successful conclusion." However, five years later the story is still the same, so that the Director's Annual Report states "intensive activities were under way in the Southern Department in locating and treating an estimated 300 cases of yaws which were expected to be the last, and which should be eliminated early in 1960." No cases were found in other parts of the Island. Unfortunately, cases were still being discovered and in 1961, 33 were diagnosed as being yaws. Of these, only one was from the Southern Department, while there were 14 each from the Northern and Western Departments, and four from the Northwestern—areas from which the disease was thought to have been cleared. To find these cases nearly two and a half million people had to be screened by seven work groups. The moral of this history is first, that eradication is not an easy business at any time and that programs are apt to continue long after the anticipated date of success. Secondly, transmission is still continuing in Haiti in spite of intensive investigations, and this could be due either to the inherent difficulties in finding the last yaws' cases in the population or to introduction from other parts of South America, or theoretically by evolution from venereal syphilis by non-venereal passage through several generations of the infection. How long will it be possible to maintain these seven work teams in the field to examine repeatedly millions of people and finding only the occasional case? And what will happen when they go or are diverted to other duties? Will some yaws-like disease make a comeback or will there be a substantial increase in syphilis as the immunity of the population diminishes? We do not know the answers to these questions at this time, but at least they should be kept in mind. Two things seem advisable: that overoptimism should be avoided, and some degree of surveillance will be necessary for a long time to come.*

Pinta

With pinta, the outlook does not seem uncertain, for the organism differs considerably from the yaws-syphilis one. So far the pinta treponeme has not been adapted to growth in any animal apart from man, which alone serves to distinguish it from the others of the group. The organisms of yaws and syphilis are so much alike that there is no certain way of telling which is which in the laboratory. There are three stages of the disease in pinta: the first being the primary sore on some piece of exposed skin, the next being the more extensive blue pigmentation of the skin, and the final one being a non-infectious stage in which the blueness disappears and only permanent white scars remain. The disease is very chronic so that the blue stage, in which the infected skin is teeming with treponemes, may last for many years. Diagnosis is easy for there is nothing else like it; people come forward willingly for treatment, for it is very disfiguring; and the response to penicillin is prompt. All these factors make it probable that pinta will be wiped out in the not too far distant future. The importation from abroad is not a problem, since the disease exists only in Central America. The chances for the organisms re-evolving from other treponemes are remote since they are so substantially different.

The Future

Attempts to predict the future are usually not worth-while. In spite of this, I will try to project the ideas in the chapter into the next 50 years, the assumption being made that the economic progress will be such that the world by that time will have reached a standard of living comparable at least to that now enjoyed by the United States.

In 50-years' time, pinta will have long since vanished, wiped out by

* The Yaws Eradication program in Haiti is now being terminated and no longer exists as a separate entity in that country. Progressive integration of its staff and program into the National Health Services was commenced in 1962. The program has had a dramatic success; in the 1940's perhaps 60 per cent of the rural population of Haiti was thought to be infected, while in 1962 only 15 yaws cases could be discovered after a final mass screening. However, the population probably still contains a small number of yaws cases. It will be interesting to see in the next decade or two whether the infection will flare up again either from this small residual seeding, or from importation from abroad, or by evolution from syphilis spread by non-venereal means.

eradication programs. Yaws and non-venereal syphilis will have been reduced almost to the vanishing point by a combination of antibiotic therapy, improved hygiene, and the wearing of clothes. Syphilis will still exist but in a very modified form. If present trends continue, sexual intercourse between both unmarried members of the opposite sex and those of the same sex will become much more accepted by society, so that promiscuity will prevail in an ever-widening fashion. This will lead to much more frequent transmission of treponemes and the selection of increasingly "acute" forms of the disease as described in Theory 4. However, the improved care of the pregnant mother may cut down sharply on the number of congenital infections so that the more serious internal lesions of syphilis may largely disappear. What will be left in 50-years' time will be a rapidly transmitted infection, spread venereally, and not much more serious than the common cold is today.

REFERENCES

1. COCKBURN, T. A.: The origin of the treponematoses. W.H.O. Bulletin, 1961.
2. VELDKAMP, H.: Isolation and characteristics of *Treponema zuelzerae* nov. species. and anaerobic free-living Spirochaete. Antonie Leeuwenhoek, 1960, **26:** 103–25.
3. DE BRUIJN, J. H.: Serological relationship between *Treponema zuelzerae* and the Reiter strain of *T. pallidum*. Antonie Leeuwenhoek, 1961, **27:** 98–102.
4. D'ALESSANDRO, G., ZAFFIRO, P., AND DARDONAI, L.: *On the Antigenic Structure of Treponema pallidum*. Presentation at World Forum, Washington, D.C., 1962 (to be published).
5. FERRIS, G. F.: *The Sucking Lice*. San Francisco. Pacific Coast Entomological Soc., Calif. Acad. Sci., 1951.
6. POLLOCK, J. S. M.: Sibbens or sivvens—the Scottish yaws. Trans. Roy. Soc. Trop. Med. & Hyg., 1953, **47:** 431–36.
7. MEANS, P. A.: *Ancient Civilization of the Andes*. Scribner, New York, 1942.
8. MOONEY, J.: *Aboriginal Population of America*. Smithsonian Institution (Misc. Coll. No. 7), Washington, D.C., 1928.
9. ELIAS, NORBERT: *Über den Prozess der Zivilisation*. Verlag hans zum Falken, Basel, 1939.
10. SALZMAN, L. F.: *English Life in the Middle Ages*. Oxford Univ. Press, Oxford, 1926.
11. COULTON, G. G.: *Social Life in Britain from the Conquest to the Reformation*. Cambridge Univ. Press, Cambridge, 1918.
12. A Task Force Report to the Surgeon General, U.S.P.H.S., on Syphilis Control in the United States. U.S.P.H.S., Washington, D.C., 1962.
13. ANDREWS, J. M. AND LANGMUIR, A. D.: The philosophy of disease eradication. Amer. J. Public Health, 1963, **53:** 1–21.
14. COCKBURN, T. A., AND MACLEOD, K. I. E.: Venereal disease survey in Cincinnati. Cincinnati J. Med., 1963, **44:** 81–83.
15. COCKBURN, T. A.: Syphilis in Cincinnati. Cincinnati J. Med., 1962, **43:** 361–63.

CHAPTER 8

Cholera

CHOLERA IN ITS pandemic form is a very new disease, dating back only as far as 1817. In that year it appeared for the first time in Calcutta and quickly made its way around the world. Four times in the nineteenth century it broke out of its home in Bengal in India in this fashion to reach almost to the fartherest limits of human societies. Finally, modern science was able to devise means of holding it in check, but even now it remains a constant threat, as has been vividly illustrated in the past year by the appearance of new epidemics in the Far East, particularly in the Philippines. A related infection called paracholera is endemic in Indonesia, but the connection between these two types is not very clear at the moment. An excellent review of the literature on all aspects of the disease has been compiled by Pollitzer (1).

By what means did this new disease appear? And how do we know that it is a new disease? It seems that something like it had already been present in India and the Dutch East Indies before 1817, but in a form that did not have the tremendous capacity for spread possessed by the present type. Pollitzer quotes a number of instances prior to 1817 in which a disease resembling cholera was described by physicians, and which is usually accepted as substantial evidence that it was well established before making its debut as a world traveler. Yet cholera is not always an easy disease to diagnose, and some of those early epidemics could as well have been due to dysentery organisms as due to the cholera vibrios. In 1959–60, I was called in as consultant to an epidemic in Karachi that was labeled as cholera. There were several hundred cases reported, and special wards were opened in a hospital in the city to accommodate them. Now dysentery was an everyday event there at that time, especially among the refugees from the partition of India who were living in poverty and squalor in various shanty towns around the city. Undoubtedly many of the cases labeled cholera in 1959–60 were not cholera but dysentery; in fact I myself did not see a typical case during my stay there. There were plenty of patients who were very ill, and some had very watery stools, but entirely lacking were those patients with extreme dehydration and typical rice water stools so commonly seen in East Pakistan. The matter was confused by the isolation of vibrios from two or three of the patients. In the Indian subcontinent it is normal to recover such organisms from a percentage of healthy persons, and it is very difficult to tell whether or not these are pathogenic. If the diagnosis can be so difficult at times today, then the precise interpretation of descriptions of two hundred years ago can be impossible.

Yet it is likely that a form of cholera did exist before 1817. The alternative would be to accept that either a free-living form suddenly became a violent pathogen, or that a harmless saprophyte quickly became a killing organism. Therefore, it is accepted here that some of the old descriptions did in fact apply to epidemics of cholera. The question now is how this old form arose and what gave it its capacity for transcontinental spread at the beginning of the nineteenth century.

In previous papers (2, 3) the suggestion has already been made that the cholera vibrio is descended from those vibrios free living in water, particularly those found in the ponds or "tanks" of surface water in Bengal. Over the millenia, persons drinking this water must have been infected with these, and so in time have acquired as saprophytes some strains descended from individual organisms preadapted to life in the human intestine. As the population of Bengal increased and there was more rapid passage of the organisms from one human intestine to another, some strains with pathogenic qualities would be selected. With the coming of the British in the later part of the seventeenth century, and the foundation of Calcutta with its numerous millions and lack of sanitation, this process of natural selection of the pathogenic forms would be hastened. The key position of Calcutta on the trade routes of the world would complete the picture, and cholera would be launched on its career as a pandemic disease.

It is well known that vibrios closely resembling the one causing cholera are numerous in waters in many parts of the world. They are also frequent in marine and river animals; indeed the most widely-held theory among Bengali physicians is that cholera is brought up the Ganges in the dry weather by a certain kind of fish. This fish is easy to catch during the cholera season, and in its intestines vibrios resembling those of cholera can be found.

Of course, the conditions in Bengal are not unique; they are found also in the deltas of many large rivers. In such places vibrios would be expected to evolve pathogenic strains from free-living forms, and possibly the paracholera of Indonesia arose also in this fashion.

The epidemiology of the epidemic type of infection was clearly worked out, many years ago, spreading along the trade and pilgrim routes through the agencies of bad hygiene, polluted water, flies, and overcrowding. The most significant feature of the nineteenth-century pandemics was that they died away, leaving no permanent foci outside Asia. In the twentieth century, the Asian foci rapidly dwindled down to one or two sharply localized areas. Today, the disease does not appear to exist in Russia or China (personal communication from Prof. B. H. Pastukhov of the 1958 Soviet Medical Mission to East Pakistan) or in Japan, the Philippines, Indonesia, or Ceylon, except when introduced from outside. The outbreak of paracholera of 1961 involved many countries of the Far East and apparently began in China. Most countries affected had had no such disease for many years. In Thailand, cholera appears for about three years at a time, but then is not seen for five or seven years. It is not known whether the infection is endemic there or is repeatedly reintroduced. The only place where it has been found with regularity all the year round, year after year, decade after decade, has been the Indian subcontinent.

At the beginning of the twentieth century, cholera seems to have been endemic in Burma, Bengal, and on the east coast of India near the sea and associated with rivers. However, in the course of 50 years, the geographic distribution of the endemic infection has progressively dwindled so that today, although the epidemic type is still likely to appear in most parts, only Bengal remains a permanent focus. Further research may show that cryptic or undiagnosed cholera is present in all seasons and years in places like Burma, Nepal, and Thailand; but until this has been demonstrated, Bengal must be regarded as the primary source of all epidemics. Therefore, should the infection be eliminated from Bengal, it would almost certainly disappear from the world.

The main epidemiological features of endemic cholera have been long known, with some of the original observations dating back nearly a century. By the end of the nineteenth century, the areas of endemicity had been clearly defined, the nature of the countryside in which it was found was described, the relationship of the disease to the weather, especially the monsoon, had been noted, and the inability of *Vibrio cholerae* to survive for long periods in water containing large numbers of competing organisms and the potentialities of the village tanks or ponds of surface water in spreading infection had been observed. The fact that the cholera vibrio could withstand a very high pH had been discovered and indeed utilized in isolating the organism in pure culture.

However, efforts to provide an explanation for these features have so far been unsuccessful. During 1958–60, I re-examined and confirmed some of these epidemiological features and offered a theory and supporting data to explain them (2).

The theory presented here is that the tanks of water are, in fact, the main means of spread of the infection; the seasonal fluctuations of the disease and possibly the limitations of the endemic area are the results of fluctuations in the pH of the tank water. Examination of a number of tanks over a period of a year has shown that in sunny weather the pH commonly rises from about 7.0–7.5 in the morning to as high as 10.0 and occasionally to 10.5 in the afternoon. But when it rains, this rise is prevented, and the pH may fall below 7.0. These fluctuations are the result of the activity of the algae in the water which liberate either carbon dioxide or oxygen according to the intensity of the light available. This range of pH's would give an advantage to the vibrio in the water over other intestinal organisms and permit them to survive, and, through natural selection, may have been responsible for producing the alkaline-resisting capacities of the organism.

The Endemic Area

Bengal is mainly the land formed by the Ganges-Brahmaputra Delta. In the 1947 partition, it was divided between India and Pakistan, and the eastern half is now East Pakistan. Ecologically, the two sides differ significantly; West Bengal has an enormous urban population centered in Calcutta, while East Pakistan is one of the most rural countries in the world. There are only two large towns in East Pakistan, Dacca with about 600,000 population and Chittagong with 300,000 and these have reached these proportions only since partition. So far as the cholera vibrio is concerned, Bengal must be regarded as one unit, for considerable numbers of people, presumably carrying with them the causal organisms of the disease, still move across the border.

Calcutta was founded by the British in the eighteenth century. It is a great, sprawling slum with most unhygienic conditions. The overcrowding is gross, and every night large numbers of people sleep in the streets and in the railway stations. Poverty is everywhere, and beggars are numerous. Half of the water supply is simply untreated crude river water. The river itself is highly polluted, and the cholera vibrio has been found in it at most times of the year.

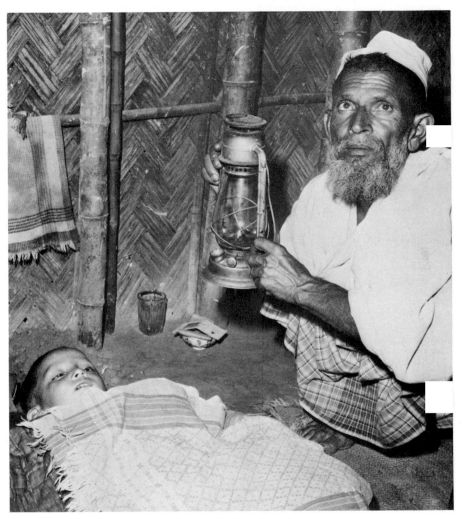

Plate I. Cholera in Bengal.

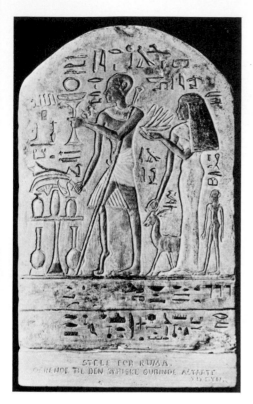

STELE FOR RUMA.
OFFERING TIL DEN SYRISKE GUDINDE ASTARTE

Plate II. The oldest representation of crippling probably due to poliomyelitis is the funerary slab of the Egyptian Rem, or Roma, sculptured more than 3,000 years ago. Rem is identified only as a "doorkeeper." He walks with a stick because his right leg is shortened and its muscles are atrophied, resulting in *pes equinovarus*. With his wife and son he is sacrificing to Astarte, perhaps in the hope that the boy will not contract the dread disease.
Carlsberg Glyptothek, Copenhagen. *Photograph courtesy of The National Foundation.*

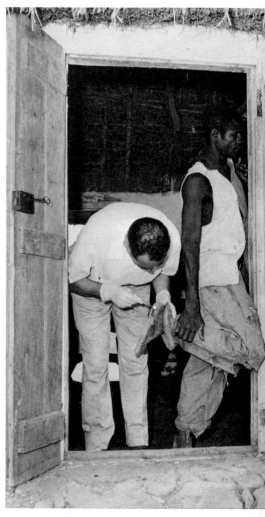

Plate III. "Show your feet" is the order of the day in Haiti, where, with the assistance of the Pan American Sanitary Bureau and the United Nations International Children's Emergency Fund (UNICEF), the government is carrying out a program to eradicate yaws. Signs of the infection are frequently found on the feet. UNICEF contributes equipment and supplies, while technical advisory services are provided by the Pan American Sanitary Bureau, executive body of the Pan American Health Organization and regional office of the World Health Organization. (Pan American Health Organization)

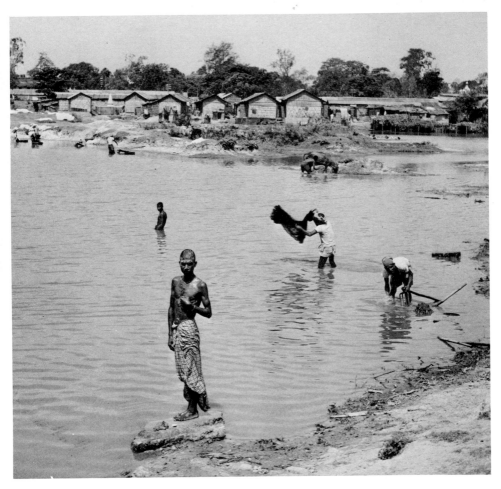

Plate IV.   Morning at a tank near Dacca, East Pakistan. Men bathe, clean a plough, throw a fishnet. In the background, dhobies wash clothes, man washes a bullock. In the far distance is a row of latrines.

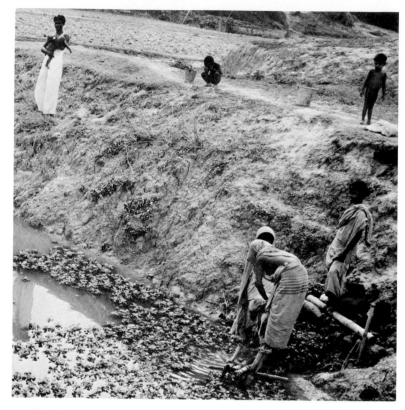

Plate V. Woman drawing water at a tank as her family waits on the bank.

Plate VI. At a roadblock in Comilla, all passers-by are vaccinated against smallpox.

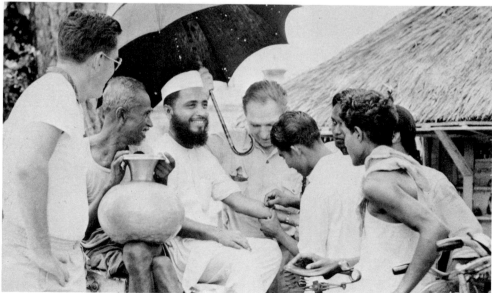

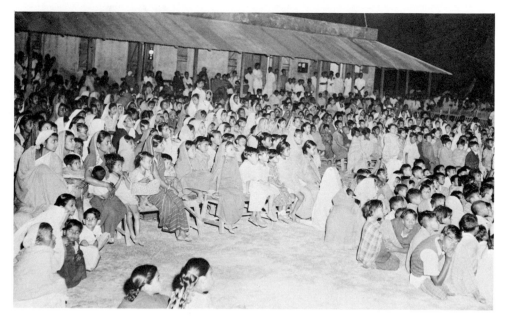

Plate VII. A crowd of 2,000 women and children saw a health show in a village near Comilla, East Pakistan. Health shows were used to further a mass vaccination campaign during the 1958 smallpox epidemic. About 30 million Pakistanis were inoculated.

Plate VIII. Lady volunteers in Khulna, East Pakistan, trained in the technique of smallpox vaccination. In countries that have the purdah system, male technicians cannot vaccinate women, and professional women health workers are very scarce.

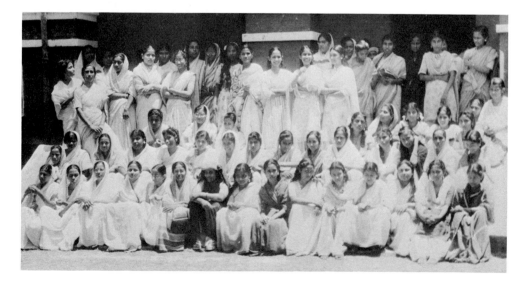

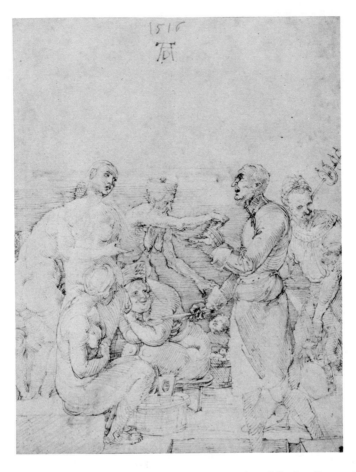

Plate IX.   "Women's Public Bath" by Albrecht Dürer, Devonshire Collection, Chatsworth.
Reproduced by permission of the Trustees of the Chatsworth Settlement.

Dürer found his best opportunities in sketching nude women at the public baths and made a series of drawings. In this particular drawing it will be noted that the women are displaying no modesty about the artist sketching them nor the men selling food and drinks.

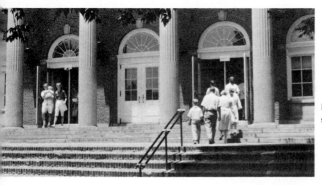

Plate X. No queues—just a steady stream in and out.

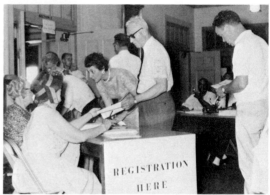

Plate XI. One doctor and fifteen volunteers can supply twelve thousand people in six hours.

Plate XIII. HQ in City Hall. Dr. Albert B. Sabin.

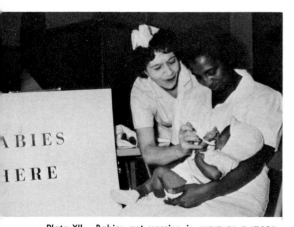

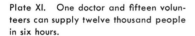

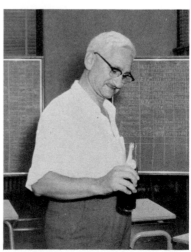

Plate XII. Babies get vaccine in syrup on a spoon.

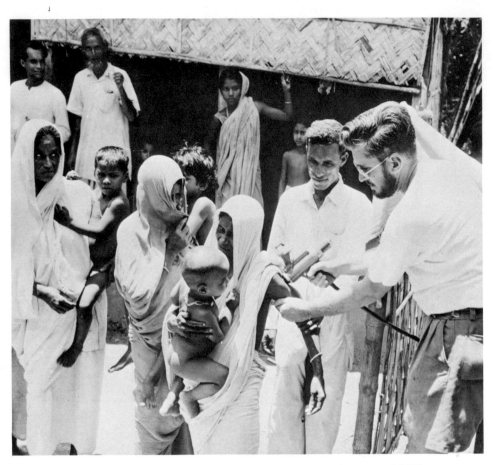

Plate XIV.   The Hypospray Jet Injector delivering cholera shots at the rate of 6,000 per day in East Pakistan. With this injector, Mr. Richard Towle, International Cooperation Administration, with two Pakistani assistants, can keep pace with more than a dozen teams of doctors, nurses, sterilizers, and assistants who use only needles and syringes.

East Pakistan is different. Here, about 45 million people, more than 95 per cent of the population, live in small communities, each with its own farming area. Some have only a few individuals of one family, while others may house several hundred persons. Where the land is most suitable for farming, the communities are smaller and only a hundred yards or so apart; where flooding is frequent, they are farther apart and larger. Since each group of houses is hidden by trees and surrounded by apparently empty fields of rice and jute, at first sight the countryside seems almost uninhabited; in reality it is one of the most heavily populated areas of the world, with nearly 1,000 persons per square mile.

The land is flat and only a few feet above sea level. Dacca Airport, about 100 miles from the sea, is 24 feet above sea level, and much of the coastal area is actually below the high-tide level, being protected by a system of dikes. The heavy rainfall of the monsoon and the huge masses of water pouring down the Ganges and Brahmaputra Rivers cause extensive flooding, and in most years about one-third of the land disappears under water. In real flood years, such as 1954, the larger portion of the delta area is submerged.

The inhabitants have become adapted to life under these conditions during many centuries. To cope with the floods, each hamlet or village has been built on a mound. The holes in the ground made by digging soil for these mounds are the tanks, and each village is usually surrounded by a number of them. In dry weather these tanks are the source of the water for the community, and a center of social life. Everyone visits them daily to wash clothes, for abiutions, to swim, to collect water for drinking and cooking, to fish, or to wash a cow or a buffalo. Sometimes there is a latrine perched on one end, and commonly, when it rains, the surface water from the houses flows into the tanks.

The houses are usually clean, with polished beaten mud and dung floors and little refuse lying around. Flies are not a major problem except around cattle sheds, and in the monsoon they are almost absent. Each family stores the year's supply of rice in large pots. After the monsoon starts in July, the mounds with their dwellings stick above the water like little islands. Nearly all roads disappear, and the villagers travel by their boats, which during the dry weather have been lying submerged in the tanks. At any time the rivers are the main highways of the Eastern Province, but during the monsoon almost everything travels by water. Water transport by sail or oar is slow, and 10 miles can be a hard day's journey. North of Dacca, the land rises slightly and is more heavily wooded, so that these conditions are found usually only along the rivers.

Patterns of Occurrence

In Bengal cholera occurs all the year round, in both the rural areas and Calcutta. Calcutta has long been the industrial and commercial heart of Bengal, and every day tens of thousands of people from the rural areas pour into it, although since partition those from East Pakistan have been diverted to Dacca. Since the infection is, without doubt, endemic in the rural areas, almost every day the vibrio must be reintroduced into Calcutta and Dacca.

Many years ago a number of workers delineated the extent of the rural endemic area in Bengal. It consisted of the coastal region and extended inland to include Rajshahi District. North of that, cases of cholera were numerous, but only in the dry season. This situation is much the same today. In Figure 7, based on the weekly reports of the Province's Directorate of Health Services, the districts of East Pakistan are marked according to the proportion of weeks in which cholera was reported over a four-year period. About 150 miles inland, parallel to the coast, but now south of Rajshahi, there is a clear line of demarcation. North of this endemic borderline cholera is reported in the dry season only, 40 per cent of the total weeks or less. South of it, the disease occurs 70 to 100 per cent of the weeks, or all year round when allowance is made for the deficiencies of the reporting system (Figure 6).

On a map of the Province marked with 250-foot contours, the endemic and non-endemic areas seem to be identical except for some slightly higher ground north of Dacca and the range of hills to the east. However, in this flat land even a few feet make a big difference, and in general, except for the land along the river bottoms, the terrain rises gently to the north of the endemic borderline; south of it the land is universally flat and barely above sea level. This affects drainage, for as described by Macnamara (1), the water in the endemic area is almost stationary in the dry season.

The spread of cholera in the rural area differs from that in the city, for there is little overcrowding in the small hamlets except during the monsoons. There is also a relatively large degree of isolation between the tiny communities, since the women are in purdah and seldom leave the home, and most travel is on foot or by the slow-moving boat. Except for the tanks and the methods of excreta dis-

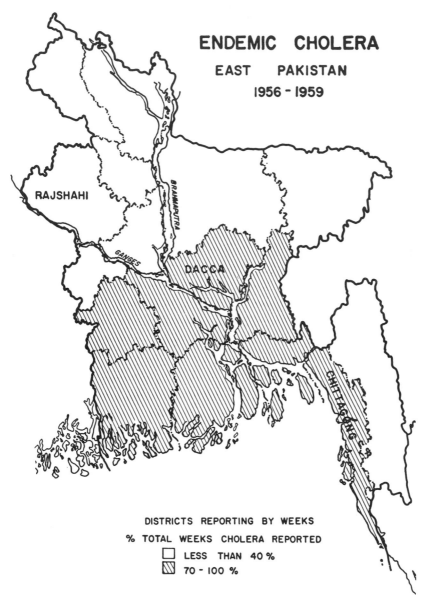

ENDEMIC CHOLERA

EAST   PAKISTAN

1956 - 1959

RAJSHAHI

BRAHMAPUTRA

GANGES

DACCA

CHITTAGONG

DISTRICTS REPORTING BY WEEKS

% TOTAL WEEKS CHOLERA REPORTED

☐ LESS THAN 40 %

▨ 70 - 100 %

Figure 6. Percent of 208 weeks when cases of cholera were notified, by district, East Pakistan, 1956–59. No districts reported cases for 40–70 per cent of the total weeks.

posal, the hygiene of the communities is of a fairly high standard.

It was Koch who first suggested that the tanks might be the most important means of spread, and many other workers have agreed with him. When the whole population washes in the water used for drinking and cooking, there must be a communal sharing of intestinal organisms. Most communities have isolated and screened latrines, but sometimes these are perched on the edge of the tanks, so that the water is further polluted. Toward the end of the dry season in April and May, the water has sunk to a low level and become stagnant and unpleasant. Beyond doubt, the tank is the greatest means of spreading the cholera vibrio during the greater part of the year. However, it is not the only means. The factors of personal contact, flies, and infected food still play a part, if only a minor one, especially in the larger villages, the overcrowded and insanitary "old" towns of Dacca and Chittagong, and in the crowded trains and other public transport systems.

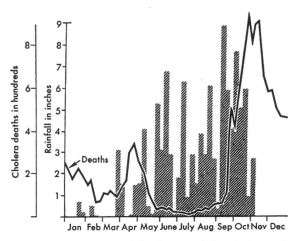

Figure 7. Rainfall in Dacca and deaths from cholera in East Pakistan, by week, 1959. *Note:* The lag in case reporting of deaths may be as much as two weeks.

That the tanks are closely implicated in the spread of infection is indicated by the epidemiology of the infection in the endemic areas. There are two kinds of occurrences. In the first, only one or two persons, usually small children, become ill in a village; in the second, 20 or 30 persons acquire cholera within one or two days and then only a few more, indicating an explosive common-source infection. The former type of outbreak is probably expressive of the immunity status of the village, in which only the small children are still susceptible, while the latter can be explained best on the basis of some vehicle of spread common to everyone, such as the tank water.

Traditionally, the cholera season ends with the onset of the monsoon (Figure 7). The abatement of local epidemics whenever a heavy, unseasonable rainfall occurred in the dry season of 1958 has been described elsewhere (2).

The influence of temperature has been less well recognized. When deaths from cholera in East Pakistan are averaged over a five-year period, a smaller cholera cycle during the winter months can be recognized in addition to the major cycle during the dry months (Figure 8). As the days grow shorter and colder, cholera diminishes,

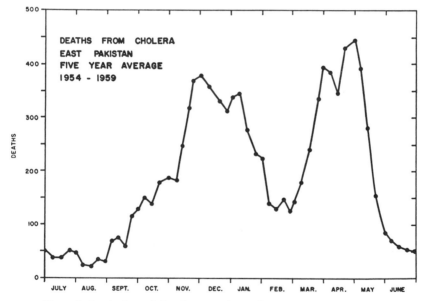

Figure 8. Deaths from cholera in East Pakistan, by month, 1954–59 average.

although there is some lag from the fall peak in November and December. Rainfall, sunshine, and temperature data are given in Table 14. The peak periods for cholera are in the hot months of the year when there is no rain.

Two exceptional years in the past decade were 1953 and 1954. In 1953 the monsoon finished earlier than usual, the cholera season started sooner, and the incidence was higher than normal. In 1954, flooding was extensive, largely due to unusually heavy flows down the Brahmaputra. Most of the delta was under water, some of it for as long as three months. During that time cholera was at a particularly low level for East Pakistan. Contrary to popular belief abroad, but well known in Benjal, the flood periods are freer from infectious disease than the dry periods.

TABLE 14. LENGTH OF DAY, SUNSHINE, RAINFALL, AND MEAN TEMPERATURE, BY MONTH, KHULNA, EAST PAKISTAN, 1959

Month	Day length (hours)	Sunshine (hours)	Temperature [1] (degrees Fahrenheit)	Total rainfall (inches)
January	11.00	9.57	68	0.4
February	11.25	9.34	74	1.0
March	12.00	8.00	81	1.3
April	12.40	7.55	86	3.9
May	13.10	7.10	87	7.4
June	13.30	4.43	85	12.0
July	13.25	4.52	84	14.4
August	12.55	4.01	84	13.2
September	12.20	4.88	85	8.4
October	11.40	5.70	82	5.4
November	11.05	8.82	76	1.0
December	10.50	9.03	70	.1

[1] Highest recorded, 107° F., lowest recorded, 39° F.

Source: Report on the Khulna Multipurpose Project, East Pakistan Water and Power Development Authority, 1959.

Experimental Theory

There have been many attempts to explain the epidemology of cholera by changes in the physical conditions of water, but so far none have been successful. There is no difficulty in finding the vibrio in the rivers around Calcutta or in places such as the tanks where religious washings take place, but the difficulty is in accounting for the relationship between the rainfall and temperature and the appearances of outbreaks, as well as the confinement of the endemic disease in so small an area.

The one feature that sets the vibrio apart from all other intestinal pathogens is its capability of thriving in media that are highly alkaline. The upper limits of resistance to pH do not seem to have been clearly defined, but the organism can multiply at a pH of 9.2 and probably survive for long periods at a much higher pH. Generally in biology, characteristics so marked as these are not due to chance, but are the results of intense natural selection pressures in the environment. It seemed to me that the water in the tanks might have alkalinities of a magnitude that would provide the necessary selection pressures and that the seasonal and geographic relationships of the disease could be accounted for by variations in the pH. Other workers have studied this matter, but they emphasized chiefly the river water and not the tanks, and no allowance was made for the biological activity of the algae in the water at different times of the day.

The tanks in Bengal contain so much algae that normally the water is a deep green color when it is not muddied. The concentration of algae and the rate of photosynthesis at any given time are the result of a highly complex interplay of many factors, but the major ones are the amount of organic and inorganic matter in the water and the amount of light available. Related to the photosynthesis, but not proportional to it (4), is the respiration of water plants. Since the rate of photosynthesis is normally faster than the rate of respiration, in day-

TABLE 15. RELATIONSHIP OF pH TO THE DEATH RATE OF SALMONELLA (EBERTHELLA) TYPHI AT 20° C

pH	3.8	5.0	5.4	6.4	7.1	7.6	8.7	9.5
Half-life (hours)	0.28	23.0	27.0	21.0	6.8	2.7	1.4	1.0

Source: Cohen, B.: Disinfection Studies. J. Bact., 1922, 7:183–230.

light these plants absorb carbon dioxide from and liberate oxygen into the water. At night the reverse process takes place. Also, photosynthesis is inhibited by too much sunlight. Beyond the optimum, the rate of activity falls rapidly, so that in bright light the maximum respiration of the algae will take place not at the surface of the water but deeper down, and in shallow surface water this factor might be of importance.

Since the endemic areas are closely linked to lands very little above sea level, and the vibrio is known to have a salt requirement, a brief exploratory study was made to see if the endemicity could be linked to the salinity of the water.

It is well known that the cholera vibrio does not live long in river water such as that of the Ganges and Nile or in sewage, and the usual explanation is that in such places it cannot cope with the competition of other organisms. In Bengal, if it could be shown that tank water has a high pH, the situation would be reversed, for intestinal organisms such as *Salmonella typhi* would soon die off (Table 15), and the cholera vibrio would survive. Should testing of surface waters in other parts of the world reveal different pH levels, an explanation would be provided for the limitation of the endemic area to small parts of Asia.

However, when heavy rain muddies and dilutes the tank water and the sky is overcast with thick clouds, the pH might not rise, and the cholera vibrio would then lose its advantage in survival. If such a situation could be shown to exist, then a reasonable explanation could be given for the well-known phenomenon of the disappearance of cholera during the monsoon.

Cholera diminishes regularly almost every year in the winter months when little or no rain falls (Figure 8). This dwindling of cases could possibly be caused by variations in the pH due to a drop in temperature, shorter days, and fewer hours of sunlight per unit of water surface area.

Collection of Samples

Therefore, it was decided in 1959 to test six tanks in the Motijheel area of Dacca for one year to see how the pH of their waters varied during changing climatic conditions and to attempt to correlate these changes with the general incidence of cholera.

The tanks were typical of those throughout the Province, except that people did not drink so much from them, since piped water was available. The people used all the tanks for washing clothes, ablutions, swimming, and fishing (Plates IV, V). Professional dhobies washed clothes in tanks 1 and 2; bullocks and buffaloes were often cleaned in tank 2; 3 had a latrine on one edge; and tanks 3, 4, 5, and 6 were close to houses whose drainage had access to the tanks. Tanks 1 and 2 were open to the sun from sunrise to sunset, while the others had a varying number of one- or two-storied houses or shacks and an occasional tree close to them. The tanks ranged in size from 50 by 100 yards to 100 by 200 yards and in depth from 4 to 18 feet.

Samples of water were usually collected from the six tanks every Monday. The water was taken from the same spot every time and from about 6 inches under the surface. Most of the time, specimens were taken three times in the day, at 5:30 to 5:45 A.M., at 11:30 to 11:45 A.M., and at 3:30 to 3:45 P.M. In a series of more intensive investigations, two of the tanks with the largest ranges of pH were sampled six times in the day at two-hour intervals beginning at 5:30

A.M. During the summer, it was daylight at 5:30, but dark during the winter.

The 5:30 A.M. specimens were kept in the dark until the laboratory opened at 8:00 A.M.; the others were all tested within half an hour of collection. Attempts were made to test water outside Dacca, especially in the non-endemic areas. After sensitive paper proved unreliable in determining the pH, a portable pH meter was used to test water on a trip to the southern end of the endemic area.

Analytical Procedures

The analytical determinations were made in the Dacca laboratory of the Ralph M. Parsons Co., of Los Angeles, Calif., which, under an ICA contract, collects data needed for its design of water supply and sewage disposal systems for Dacca and Chittagong. This laboratory is equivalent in scope and equipment to public health laboratories in the United States. After completion of the contract, the laboratory will become the nucleus of the water and sewage section of the new public health laboratory for East Pakistan. The initial specimens were tested by Dr. Gordon E. Mau, and the later ones by Jack R. Snead, both of the Parsons firm.

The procedures followed in this laboratory are those of the 10th edition of *Standard Methods for the Examination of Water, Sewage, and Industrial Waste*. Precision and accuracy of analytical results are maintained by having each chemist periodically run a quantitative analysis of an unknown synthetic sample. Any errors reported are called to the attention of the analyst, and after the cause of the errors has been determined, the previously submitted data are either corrected or discarded. From these continuous checks, it is believed that the reported data are accurate to ±5 per cent of the reported values.

Findings

The year 1959 was atypical so far as the weather was concerned. Normally, there is some light rain in January and severe wind storms with occasional rain in April, but in 1959 heavy showers occurred frequently between January and June. During the monsoon which was expected to start in June, there were often intervals of many days when no rain fell or only a little during the night. The apparent result of the unusual rains was that the anticipated epidemic

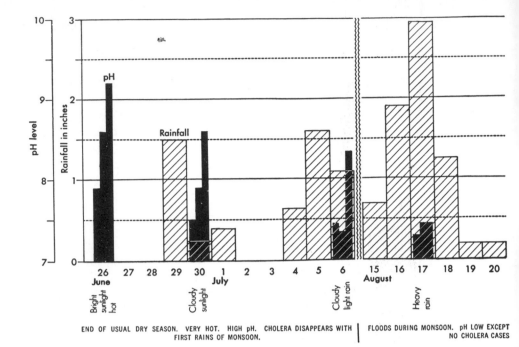

END OF USUAL DRY SEASON. VERY HOT. HIGH pH. CHOLERA DISAPPEARS WITH FIRST RAINS OF MONSOON. | FLOODS DURING MONSOON. pH LOW EXCEPT NO CHOLERA CASES

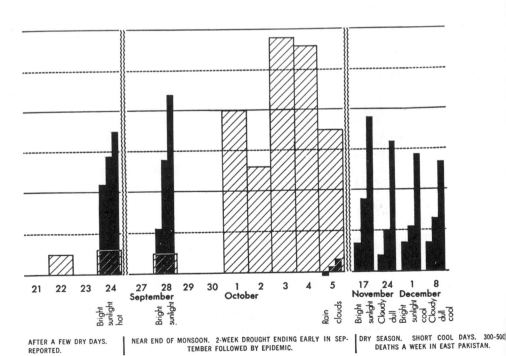

AFTER A FEW DRY DAYS. REPORTED. | NEAR END OF MONSOON. 2-WEEK DROUGHT ENDING EARLY IN SEPTEMBER FOLLOWED BY EPIDEMIC. | DRY SEASON. SHORT COOL DAYS. 300-500 DEATHS A WEEK IN EAST PAKISTAN.

Figure 9. Average of the pH levels of six tanks, Dacca, East Pakistan, 1959.

peak of April and May did not materialize on the usual scale, while perhaps as a result of the light monsoon, the cholera started earlier and more heavily in September, with deaths reaching nearly 1,000 per week. The data are given in Figure 7, which shows deaths for the whole Province but the rainfall only for Dacca. The abnormal rainfall also made more difficult the obtaining of clear-cut results with regard to the pH and its relation to sunlight and rainfall.

Samples of the relationship between the pH, the rainfall, sunlight, and time of day at four different periods of the year are given in Figures 9 and 10. At sunrise, the pH is usually quite low, being

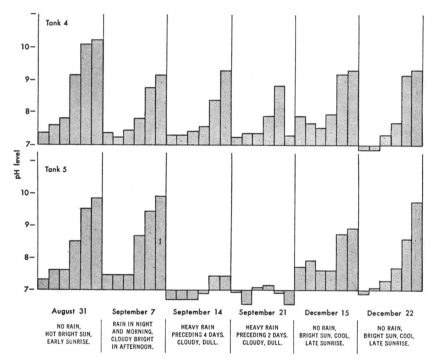

Figure 10. Studies of the pH in tanks 4 and 5, Dacca, East Pakistan, 1959. Specimens collected at 2-hour intervals, starting at 5:30 A.M.

either a little above or below 7.0, but on clear days with bright sunlight it is often above 9.0 by noon, and it can reach as high as 10.5 by late afternoon. A similar daily summer rise in the pH of a spring-fed pool with abundant Chara fragilis was observed in 1928 in the United States (5).

However, when the heavy rain, normal for the monsoon, falls either on the day of sampling or for some days before it, the pH does not rise much above 7.0 and on occasion may fall below it.

In winter, the pH still can rise to high levels, but not quite so high as during dry spells in the hot weather. Also the number of hours when this happens is much shorter than in summer when there is no rain. During a long, hot, rainless summer day the pH is above 9.0 for at least six hours, but it is at that height for only four hours in winter.

Toward the end of the monsoon in 1959, a sharp epidemic of cholera occurred in Dacca District and in the city itself. It was reported to have started the week ending September 25, but when the time lag in case reporting, which can be as much as two weeks, and the incubation period of the disease are taken into account, the date when the population first became generally infected is advanced two or three weeks to about the beginning of September. This can be related to two comparatively dry, hot, and sunny weeks beginning on August 19, when the pH of the tank water was regularly at a high level for many hours a day. The sunny period was followed by heavy rains, including five inches on September 12, and when the water was tested on September 14, the pH was about 7.0 (Figures 9 and 10). The epidemic disappeared soon after, although sporadic cases at the rate of about five or six a day continued to be admitted to the hospital in Dacca.

Observations of tanks in other parts of the endemic area were not so complete as those in Dacca, but, in general, the findings were much the same. All tanks had abundant algae except one near the town of Khulna which did not show a rise in pH. In Khulna District many tanks were surrounded by trees and shaded for most of the day, and they showed little rise in pH above 8.0.

Estimates of chloride content of water showed no differences among the surface water near the sea at Barisal and Khulna, the study area at Dacca, and Rajshahi. In general the ranges were low, between 15 and 30 mg. per liter; tank 3 which had a latrine perched on one side consistently had a content of 50–60 mg. per liter. Other data on the chemistry of the tank water in Dacca are given in Table 16. The water is very lightly buffered so that relatively large shifts in the pH can be easily attained. The chloride levels are low, which could be of significance in view of the requirements of the vibrio in culture.

The turbidity is high compared with that of river water. In December when the testing was done there is little flow in the rivers, consequently little mud, and the turbidity is about 30. The difference in turbidity is due almost entirely to the fact that tank water is full of algae and river water is comparatively free of it, which would explain why earlier observers, who tested only river water, failed to find significant pH changes. During the monsoon, the river turbidity

TABLE 16. CHEMICAL ANALYSES IN MILLIGRAMS PER LITER OF TANK WATER IN DACCA, EAST PAKISTAN

	Tank number and date of sample					
Components analyzed	1 Dec. 28, 1959	2 Dec. 28, 1959	3 Jan. 5, 1960	4 Jan. 5, 1960	5 Jan. 11, 1960	6 Jan. 11, 1960
pH	7.40	7.40	7.25	7.20	7.12	8.05
Total dissolved solids	256	264	366	217	151	148
Turbidity	140	140	50	85	130	37
Total hardness as $CaCO_3$	64	42	47	62	50	30
Total alkalinity as $CaCO_3$	78	116	56	86	56	72
Ca^{++}	16.0	9.6	9.6	15.2	14.4	8.0
Mg^{++}	4.7	1.9	3.0	4.2	2.4	1.6
Na^+	22.4	39.7	15.8	20.4		28.0
K^+	16.6	4.8	9.3	11.4	9.8	6.4
Fe^{+++}	0.68	1.28	0.6	1.0	0.18	0.30
Mn^{+++}	0.00	0.00	0.00	0.00	0.00	0.00
NH_4^+	0.17	0.03	0.008	0.08	0.05	0.23
CO_3^-	0.00	0.00	0.00	0.00	0.00	0.00
HCO_3^-	47.6	70.8	34.2	52.5	34.2	43.9
$SO_4^=$	1.8	0.8	11.0	13.0	11.4	11.6
Cl^-	33.0	17.2	26.1	34.0	22.7	22.3
NO_3^-	0.16	0.05	0.42	0.22	0.44	0.44
NO_2^-	0.11	0.01	0.01	0.13	0.02	0.03
$PO_4^=$	0.05	0.04	0.02	0.06	0.34	0.12
F^-	0.10	0.05	0.10	Tr.	0.15	0.10
$SiO_3^=$	27.2	19.2	7.6	12.1	18.9	13.6
BO_2^-	6.73	10.3			13.1	4.8

due to mud is more than 300. There is no evidence of gross pollution with sewage.

Because the rate of photosynthesis depends on the intensity of sunlight, the rate varies according to the season of the year and the degree of cloudiness. However, experience shows that local factors such as the muddiness of the water, the amount of shade provided by trees and buildings, and the cover provided by water plants on the surface have considerable influence on a particular tank. For example, in most tanks the pH dropped rapidly within half an hour after sunset, but the presence of a two-story house on the west side of a tank would be the equivalent of a half-hour advance in the sunset and a shortening by that time-period of the pH peak.

In the summer, the days are longer and the period of high pH is also longer. The sun is overhead, so that each unit of water surface receives more light than in winter when the sun's rays hit the water at an angle. However, in a normal year, the summer also largely coincides with the monsoon when rain reduces the number of sunny hours each day and muddies and dilutes the water in the tanks.

Discussion

Cholera is a disease in retreat. After being spread over nearly all the world in the nineteenth century, it is now largely pinned down to a small and diminishing portion of southeast Asia. Even here, the trend in the incidence is decidedly downward, as indicated in the yearly figures for East Pakistan (Figure 11), and the shrinkng of the area where the disease is found all year round. A few decades

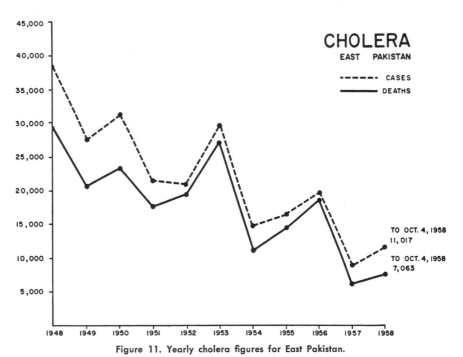

Figure 11. Yearly cholera figures for East Pakistan.

ago the endemic area included the Rajshahi District; now the area's northern boundary is about 50 miles south. However, cholera is still a serious potential threat to mankind. Deaths at a rate approaching 1,000 a week are reported at certain seasons in East Pakistan, and developments such as fast jet plane travel or the chance of a war in the region might tip the balance once again in favor of the vibrio and result in major epidemics elsewhere. Therefore, it is of importance to know the factors which influence the infection in its original, and perhaps only permanent, home.

Most studies, even the most recent (6), consider Calcutta to be the main focus of cholera. I suggest that in Bengal the endemic infection is primarily rural, and that the Calcutta urban region is of secondary importance. Many other cities in the world with large populations and overcrowding like Calcutta have experienced cholera epidemics, but in these always the infection has died out. London in the mid-nineteenth-century days of John Snow closely resembled Calcutta with its masses of people, insanitary slums, and cholera-infected river, but the vibrio failed to establish a permanent foothold. Calcutta has what the other cities do not have, a surrounding country-side in which cholera always exists.

Of course, the ecology of any infection is a highly complex affair. Variations in three main factors, the host, the pathogen, and the environment, all must be taken into account. However, there must be something special to account for the persistence of cholera in Bengal when the infection dies out so easily elsewhere. The dominant factor cannot be merely bad hygiene or polluted river water, or the infection would have persisted in many other parts of the world. The investigations reported here were limited to the endemic area of Bengal, so that it is not possible to deduce from the data that the pH of the tank water alone is responsible for the localized endemicity. To test this possibility, similar studies would have to be undertaken in areas in which cholera has never been endemic. The data do allow concluding that the pH is a factor to be taken into account. They also permit theorizing that the pH is responsible for making the tanks the main means of spread of the vibrio and provide an explanation for the connection between the incidence of the disease and the changing climatic conditions.

One can even speculate that the infection evolved in Bengal because of this factor. It is well known that vibrios morphologically similar to the cholera vibrio abound in the water of this region, and it is easy to imagine that the population became parasitized with them through drinking this water. Indeed, a main difficulty in diagnosing sporadic cases of cholera here is that a certain percentage of the population are carriers of vibrios that look like the cholera vibrio but are said to be non-pathogenic. As the population of Bengal increased, especially after the founding of Calcutta, increased passage of these could produce a strain of vibrio pathogenic to man.

If further work should confirm that cholera is endemic in Bengal because of polluted tank water, then the answer to the problem of eradication of the infection lies in the provision of pure water for the villagers. The government of East Pakistan, with the assistance of the United States through the International Cooperation Administration, is engaged in a program with a goal of one tubewell for every 400 people. About 120,000 wells are required. By the end of June 1960, 13,000 new wells were sunk and 12,000 choked-up wells rehabilitated, bringing the total of functioning wells in the Province to about 65,000. A similar program with the same target, which was set by the Bhore Commission before the partition of India, is underway in the rural areas of West Bengal. Surveys are under way in Calcutta, Dacca, and Chittagong to determine the best way of providing pure piped water supplies to those cities.

Because of the population distribution, even the achievement of this first target will not bring clean water to every villager. If cholera is to be eradicated, a special effort must be made, particularly in the endemic areas of Bengal on both sides of the border, to provide enough tubewells to reach everyone. International agencies that are interested in wiping out this disease should actively support these efforts of the local governments.

Cholera is endemic in Bengal, the major remaining focus of infection, because of polluted drinking water. The eradication of cholera from Bengal, and therefore from the world, depends largely on the success of the Pakistani and Indian governments in replacing the village tanks with a source of safe water. Should studies show paracholera in Indonesia and China to be the result of similar conditions, then it will have to be dealt with by the same means.

REFERENCES

1. POLLITZER, R.: *Cholera*. W.H.O. Monograph Series No. 43, Geneva, 1959, 1019 pp.
2. COCKBURN, T. A.: Epidemic crisis in East Pakistan, April–July 1958. Public Health Rep., 1960, **75**: 26–36.

3. COCKBURN, T. A.: A theory on endemic cholera. Public Health Rep., 1959, **76**: 791–803.

4. RYTHER, J. H.: Potential productivity of the sea. Science, 1959, **130**: 602–8.

5. MATHESON, R., AND HINMAN, E. H.: A seasonal study of the plankton of a spring-fed Chara pool versus that of a temporary to semi-permanent woodland pool in relation to mosquito breeding. Amer. J. Hyg., 1930, **11**: 174–88.

6. MINISTRY OF HEALTH: *Control of Smallpox and Cholera in India*. New Delhi, Government of India, 1959.

CHAPTER 9

Smallpox, Poliomyelitis, Malaria, and Tuberculosis

SMALLPOX

ALONG WITH MALARIA, smallpox is the second of the diseases the eradication of which has been proclaimed as an objective by the World Health Organization. This step is long overdue, and indeed it is a disgrace that so serious a disease still exists when so easy a preventative has been known for more than one and a half centuries. Vaccination may not be all that Jenner claimed for it, and in particular it does not give life-long immunity, but properly performed and with a well organized campaign, it can wipe out quickly the infection from any community. The most striking example in recent years was in Bengal, East Pakistan, in 1958, when an epidemic that had been raging for more than a year and which by May 1958 was causing about 1,500 deaths a week was quickly terminated by the mass vaccination of about 30 million out of the 46 million people in the country (1). Given good will or at least enlightened self-interest among the countries of the world, there is no reason why the last case of smallpox should not disappear within two or three years. Every year the disease exists beyond that time is a measure of the lack of accord and distrust between the nations that prevails today.

When the Eleventh World Health Assembly called for an inquiry into the possibility of eradicating smallpox from the world, a report was prepared (and presented to the Twelfth World Health Assembly) in which it was estimated that the average cost of mass vaccination through the world would be $0.10 per person vaccinated, i.e., approximately 100 million dollars for the 1,000 million persons living in the endemic areas to be covered by an eradication program. It is difficult to give world figures for smallpox eradication expenditure, mainly because the cost of the campaign in many countries is included in the general public health budget. However, a number of countries have made estimates of the cost of eradication and have requested assistance from international sources to supplement the funds available nationally. A preliminary estimate prepared by these countries shows that extra-budgetary funds required to meet additional expenditure—mostly for transport and storage equipment—would represent about 10 per cent of the total cost of the national eradication program. A sum of $10 million is therefore required for additional aid for the smallpox eradication program, representing 10 per cent of the sum of $100 million estimated in 1959 as the total cost. This is based on the assumption that most countries where the disease is endemic could themselves find 85 to 90 per cent of the cost (2).

Evolution

The relationship of smallpox virus to those of infections of animals in man's ecology is quite clear; it belongs to the group of pox viruses that includes those of cow, horse, sheep, mouse, goat, etc. The conclusion is almost inescapable that when man settled down to live in one place and all these animals came to live with him—usually in the same house—there was a general transfer of organisms between the animals. The pox virus brought in by one animal soon infected the others. Repeated passage within the host animal species brought about selections of strains adapted to those hosts and so the various members of the pox group arose. As man increased in numbers, his particular virus acquired the characteristics that we know today.

Smallpox fits the description of an "acute community infection" as given in Theories 4 and 5. The virus can, therefore, continue to survive only if a very large number of susceptibles are continually available to it, so that it must have evolved since the invention of agriculture and the domestication of animals permitted the world's population to pass beyond the size required for its continued survival.

Even today this process of acquiring pox viruses from animals continues, for milkers still get cowpox. Indeed it was this cross-infection from the cows that first led to the idea of vaccination. In Europe and England before the nineteenth century, almost everybody was infected sooner or later and had a scarred face. Only one person stood out from the rest. This was the milk maid whose face remained unscarred. And so arose the compliment "as pretty as a milkmaid." That milkmaids did not get smallpox had been folklore for centuries, and at least one farmer before Jenner tried to put the idea into practice. About 1750 a farmer from Hampshire vaccinated some people and came to London to spread the idea. However, he was not well educated and no one paid any attention to him and he returned to his farm and dropped out of sight.

Without a doubt, man is still being infected from time to time with many of these pox viruses, either by handling horses, goats, and other animals that are shedding virus, or from the mouse with ectromelia that runs around the house contaminating the environment in general and food in particular with its feces and urine. There are still many parts of this world where conditions of hygiene are such that accidental infections of this kind could be transmitted from man to man. However, such an event is becoming increasingly unlikely in this modern era, and also any new organism evolving in this way would have a stiff competition from the smallpox and vaccinia already in possession of the field and even more so from the cowpox in the hands of the vaccinator. Still, if a time were to come when smallpox were eradicated and vaccination no longer applied on a large scale, the chances of a new pox virus arising would have to be considered seriously.

Eradication

The eradication of smallpox on a world basis is technically easy, but politically, logistically, financially, and geographically difficult. Obviously, no such program is going to succeed or even start in any country where there is fighting or large-scale civil unrest, as there has been in Algeria for these past seven years, or in Tibet, the Congo, Laos, and any of the other trouble spots of the world. Yet people grow tired of fighting, and even in Algeria peace came eventually. Perhaps the time will come when the disease has been wiped out of all the major regions of the world and only a few foci will remain. Already it has gone from North America, Europe, and Russia, while India is engaged in a mass vaccination campaign for her 400 millions of people. Yet the full value of this effort is not realized so long as the people of each of the nations have to be vaccinated for a disease that no longer exists in their territories. Always there will be the risk of reinfection from the foci into the cleared areas, as was vividly illustrated in 1961 when immigrants from Pakistan to England, traveling on the latest jet planes, brought the infection with them and set off a series of outbreaks in England. The governments of the world may grow tired of the continual necessity of vaccination and dealing with such episodes and may combine to stamp out the virus from its last strongholds and so realize for the first time the full benefits of eradication.

Vaccination is not very expensive in money. As performed in the U.S., it probably costs about $2.00 per person on an average, this being done usually on an individual basis in the physicians' office. In India, where it is done by relatively unskilled vaccinators at the rate of about 50 to 100 a day and the vaccine is issued in bulk lots of about a hundred to a bottle, and the salary of the vaccinator is not more than Rs 2 a day, the cost is very much less. Still when these

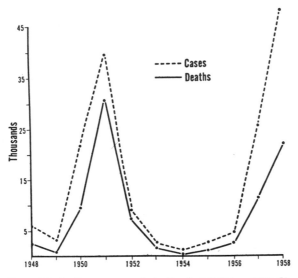

Figure 12. Smallpox cases and deaths, East Pakistan, 1948–58.

sums are translated into cost for hundreds of millions of people, they become sizable, and every year represents an undesirable drain on the economy of the world.

One of the main difficulties about vaccination is that it is usually done only half-heartedly. The person who is vaccinated only once in his life may have some residual immunity that will protect him to some extent when he becomes infected, but the mild disease that results makes him a menace to the community. He does not feel too ill to walk about and mingle with his fellows and so he spreads the virus wherever he goes. On a community scale, partial immunity is as equally undesirable. In parts of India, comparatively few have in the past been immunized between epidemics, but when the disease appears, there is a rush to be protected. This has resulted in a

cyclic state with the epidemics occurring about every five years
(Figures 12, 13,) the mass of people being protected at such times,
and then little smallpox is heard of until the immunity has decreased
and enough children born to build the required number of susceptibles for another epidemic. It is much the same pattern as in
measles except that the cycle is a little longer and the immunity is
provided not by the pathogen, but by the vaccinator. Fortunately
for the eradication programs, smallpox is a frightening disease that
terrifies persons in all countries, and vaccination is now generally
accepted (Plates VI, VII, VIII). Therefore, there is usually less diffi-

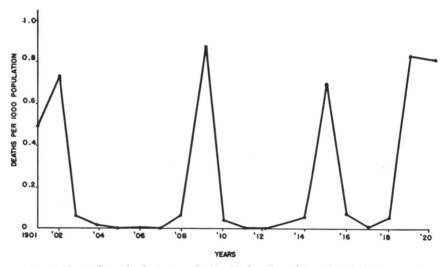

Figure 13. Smallpox deaths in Bengal 1901–20, based on data collected by Rogers (3).

culty in persuading both governments and their peoples to accept
and give active support for the programs than for most other infectious diseases.

There are still some governments that are not wholly convinced
of the need for eradication, as contrasted with control, of smallpox,
and there are still people that do not "believe" in vaccinations.
While in Swat, a small Himalayan principality on the northwest
frontiers of Pakistan and India, I found the tribesmen of this wild
and largely unpoliced land were still using variolation for protection
against smallpox and refusing to be vaccinated. They believe that
every person has to have smallpox and it is going to be difficult to
convince them to the contrary. Smallpox cults exist in various parts

of the world; for example, in India there is a hill whose rocky out-crops make it resemble a human skin with smallpox scars and rela-tives of sufferers crawl to it on their hands and knees to appease the god who has brought this misfortune on them. While serving with the British Army in West Africa during World War II as Hygiene Specialist, an epidemic was reported to have been set off by a gang of a smallpox cult. The West African cult differs from that in India in that the members of the cult apparently deliberately spread the infection in a village unless they are paid to go away. The source of their infecting matter is a body of a person dead of small-pox which is hung between two trees for several days and the liqui-fying material collected on banana leaves. This is said to be smeared on the doorways of villagers who dare defy the spirit of the disease (4).

In every continent, matters such as these will complicate the nor-mal flow of eradication events, but without doubt in the end, the disease can be wiped out completely.

While the picture of smallpox on a world scale is therefore fairly clear-cut, and all that is needed now is vigorous action, the position on a national scale during the interim, while the world eradication is progressing, is causing some headaches. Recently in 1962, a boy traveling from Brazil to Canada developed smallpox a day or so after arrival and set off a scare in New York, through which he had passed. The interesting point was that first, his vaccination certificate was not accurately completed, for the boy had not in fact been vac-cinated in Brazil. Apparently the doctor did not believe in vaccina-tion, but still signed the document. Secondly, the certificate was not adequately inspected by the quarantine officers in New York. These points illustrate the difficulties of maintaining an adequate protection to a country without great hindrance to the flow of people entering or leaving. Much the same problems have arisen in Europe in the past two years, where a huge volume of traffic has developed in the past decade from Asia and Africa. The travelers often arrive holding a piece of paper written in Urdu or Hindi which is said to be evidence of vaccination. Since the staff in Europe cannot read this, the travelers have often been passed through without comment, and the result has been a rash of small epidemics in various parts of Europe, especially in England. To many people of India, vaccina-tion using serum from a cow is a distasteful and unholy matter, so that often the tendency is to try to avoid it. There is no difficulty in finding some doctor to provide the necessary certificate without performing the vaccination. In the days of sea travel, these difficulties did not arise, since any cases developed on board ship and were recognized long before England was reached.

Vaccination is not a harmless matter. Just how many people are killed by it and how many made ill is uncertain, for the collection of the needed statistics presents many difficulties. For example, in the small epidemic in New York in 1947, a collection of data was made that indicated that 44 cases of post-vaccinial encephalitis had occurred with four deaths, and 45 cases of generalized vaccinia with two deaths. About five million people had been vaccinated (5). The difficulty with these figures is that post-vaccinial encephalitis is very hard to diagnose, since many other diseases look like it and it can follow many other infections. If five million are protected against smallpox, then in the weeks following, several cases of encephalitis could be expected to occur that would have nothing to do with the vaccination. Still the figures are in line with other experiences, including my own. In 1941–42, I was Deputy Assistant Director of Hygiene, Royal Army Medical Corps, and in charge of the hygiene of the Aldershot Command. The Command is the great peacetime base of the British Army, and in World War II was crammed tight with soldiers of all the Allied Armies. During my two years in Aldershot, more than two million British passed through the various depots there, some being fresh from civil life and others on their way abroad. All had to be vaccinated, and some of the reactions were very severe. Frequently, those being protected for the first time suffered great swelling of the arm and were off sick for a week or more. In one series of a million men of which I kept particular notice, there were four deaths from encephalitis. According to Dixon (6) post-vaccinial encephalitis ranges from an extreme of one case in a million in Gloucester, England, to one in 63 in small towns in Holland.

Public opinion in England has been turning away from mass vaccination of the general population. Vaccination had been made compulsory in 1853 at a time when smallpox was commonplace, but as time went on and the complications of the vaccination grew more troublesome than the risk of the disease, people grew irked at the necessity for the procedure. The percentage of people vaccinated grew steadily smaller, and in the 1930's, the compulsory element was repealed. At the present moment, only about 40 per cent of the population has had at least one scar. Following the recent epidemics, the matter has been brought into the open by Dick (7), who is of the opinion that general vaccination of the British population is unjustified.

According to Dick, "Probably the reported deaths from vaccination underestimated their true incidence; they were at least 15.4 per million vaccinations in the age group 0–1. The oft-repeated statement that primary vaccination after infancy was more dangerous than during infancy was also untrue, since because immunity quickly waned the risks for the latter must include the additional risks of revaccination. The mortality rate for primary vaccination in infancy plus revaccination at 15 years was 18.4 per million vaccinations, compared with a figure of 5 per million for primary vaccinations at 15 years. Further, a single vaccination in infancy did not significantly reduce the overall risk to the community, for, although it diminished the risk of contracting smallpox by 1,000-fold in the first year of life, it reduced it by only one-half at the age of 20."

Vaccination and revaccination must be done every few years to maintain a high herd immunity to smallpox, and, although it was justified for those at special risk—such as immigration and public-health officers and fever-hospital nurses—it was not for the general public. Professor Dick defined the four important points in a program which he considered would provide better protection: immigrants from endemic areas should be revaccinated 14 days before entry into Britain and should produce an adequate certificate of vaccination; control of entry of immigrants at ports should be strict; patients with smallpox should be diagnosed rapidly by a team comprising family doctor, medical officer of health, and smallpox consultant, and admitted to a smallpox, and never to a general, hospital; and there should be a thorough and scrupulous tracing and vaccination of contacts. There was no place for panic mass vaccination with all its unnecessary complications. A medical officer of health was perfectly capable of controlling a smallpox outbreak without panic.

Professor Dick considered that there were three possible policies for the future. First, we could muddle on with incomplete vaccination, and still less revaccination, with all their attendant complications and deaths. Secondly, we could try to obtain a high herd immunity; this would involve a high rate of infant vaccination, which would mean 20 babies a year being sacrificed. Even then only 10 per cent of the population would be immune at any one time. To obtain a high level of immunity in adults, revaccination would have to be repeated at least six times during life, and this would kill at least 30 persons a year and cripple another 30 from the sequelae of post-vaccinial encephalitis. Thirdly, reliance could be placed on epidemiological control as he had outlined; this method was particularly suited to an island such as Britain, where smallpox was one of the easiest diseases to control. Professor Dick added that he was a firm believer in the efficacy of smallpox vaccination when used to protect the right people at the right time; but the vast majority of people living in the United Kingdom were not at risk from smallpox, never had been at risk, and probably never would be.

I am inclined to agree with much of Dick's point of view, although his figures of the mortality from vaccination seem high to me. But what might work in a tight little island like the United Kingdom would not necessarily be practical elsewhere. It is most unlikely that such a position would be adopted in the United States. In any event the real aim is to have smallpox eradicated on a world scale, and when this is achieved, the need for vaccination anywhere will have ceased to exist.

In the past year there have been a number of pronouncements and editorials in the medical press of the United States to the effect that vaccination must be continued here. Few of these even mentioned world eradication as a solution to the problem. Surely, this is a backward way of looking at smallpox, or at the best merely an attempt to maintain the status quo. The medical professions of the Western world should be more aggressive and seek to wipe out the infection beyond the borders of their own countries. They should support and even promote such international programs, perhaps for the benefit of the infected countries, but certainly at least in the self interests of their own.

It would not be necessary for the whole world to be free of infection before the Western nations dropped the practice of universal vaccination. If only a few small foci remained in areas inaccessible by reason of backwardness, geography, or politics, a system of quarantine of unvaccinated travelers from such places would most likely be effective. Then only persons peculiarly exposed—customs officers, hospital staffs, etc.—would need protection in the remainder of the nations. Universal vaccination could then be abolished and true eradication achieved.

MALARIA

Evolution

In a preceding chapter, possible steps in the evolution of malaria have been discussed. The theories presented suggest that intracellular protozoa of the intestinal tract were carried to the liver via the portal blood system and parasitized cells there. Some of these liver parasites were liberated in the systemic blood system and were picked up by blood-sucking arthropods and so transmitted to new hosts. This would have happened long before the primates appeared on earth. The existence of mosquitoes, many tens of millions of years ago, has been very well documented, as described in Chapter 2. The principle of evolution of a parasite in parallel with its host is contained in Theory 2. These theories and facts lead to the conclusion that the early ancestral primate was already infected with malaria parasites when it first separated from other animals many millions of years ago; subsequently, as the various primate stocks split off, the parasites would accompany them and vary in parallel with their hosts. Man is quite a newcomer on earth, so that his parasites would have had less time to evolve separate features than those parasites of the lower primates, so that his plasmodia would resemble closely those of the other higher primates. Furthermore, he appeared in Africa alongside many other primates, occupying much the same habitat as they did, especially the baboons which he hunted. Therefore, there would be a continual interchange of parasites between the various species of primate and man that would prevent the selection of distinctive strains of *Plasmodium*. In his later travels over the world, he would occupy territories with monkeys and apes other than those found in Africa, and some places with no primates at all, and the scene would be set for speciation by *Plasmodium* and the appearance of the forms of human malaria parasite known to us today.

Eradication

It is against such an ecologic background that the eradication of malaria must be viewed. A decade or two ago, malaria was considered the greatest killer of man of all the infectious diseases. It was present in most places where there were anopheline mosquitoes and temperatures high enough to permit the extrinsic development of parasites. Today the position is dramatically different, for the discovery of the insecticides has placed in our hands tools that are proving highly successful in combating this infection. Many countries now report their territories to be clear of the parasite, and many of those not so successful can at least claim substantial steps in the same direction (Figure 14). The world eradication of malaria has been proclaimed as an objective by the World Health Organization and the

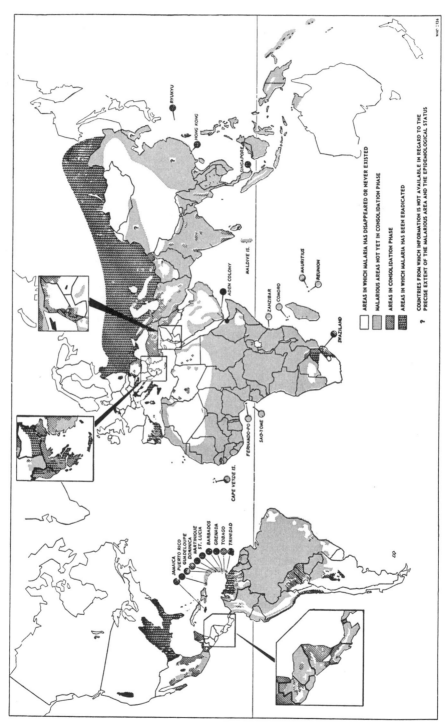

Figure 14. Malaria world situation in December 1961. (Courtesy World Health Organization)

United States, having abolished the disease from its own territory, is supporting the program with up to 50 million dollars a year.

The reason for the haste to eradicate malaria is that the insect world has displayed an unexpected capacity to develop resistance to the insecticides. Mosquitoes capable of surviving contact with the usual doses of the various kinds have been found in most parts of the world. The fear is that if malaria were merely controlled, and pushed down to a point that it was no longer a public health problem but where the parasites still existed, the time would come when it might make a comeback. The insecticide tools must be used to the maximum while they are still effective. It was on these grounds that the World Health Organization decided to recommend to the nations of the world that a major effort be made to kill off the last parasite to remove all chances of that comeback.

No one visualized the task as being easy, although some optimists talked in terms of ten years.* This optimism was partly the result of vagueness as to what was meant by eradication, for at first the concept of species eradication as applied to the plasmodium was not clearly defined, and many people still do not accept it in the form laid down in this book. There was also an underestimate of the difficulties in the field. All the difficulties of geography, logistics, politics, and personnel listed earlier have proved far greater than anticipated, so that today the programs in many countries of Africa and places like New Guinea are merely in the talking stages. Still, the program has had a very substantial success, and if it were not for the monkeys and their malaria, there would be very good hopes that at some date in the not too far distant future, the last human plasmodium would disappear. The difficulty is that it is now only too clear that monkey malaria is easily transmissible to man in the laboratory (8) and presumably also in the field. It can be passed from man to man by mosquitoes as a human infection (9). As long as the monkey infection exists there is the strong possibility that once the eradication measures are relaxed, the human population will be invaded by such monkey parasites and a fresh human strain produced.

* Just announced (Released by the U.S. Department of Health, Education, and Welfare, November 1, 1962) a successful trial of a new drug (CI501, Parke, Davis & Co.).

A single injection of a new drug given volunteers nearly a year ago is continuing to protect them from malaria induced by heavily infected mosquitoes which have been allowed to bite them at monthly intervals. Other volunteers not given the drug invariably come down with malaria after being bitten by these mosquitoes.

Providing this drug has no serious side effects, its application on a wide scale could have a profound effect upon the malaria eradication program.

There has been a tendency for malariologists to minimize the danger to their programs of possible transmission from monkeys. It is only as formidable evidence is accumulating through transmission experiments on human volunteers that reluctantly the idea is being accepted as a distinct possibility. As recently as 1961, the Expert Committee of the World Health Organization was downgrading the dangers of monkey malaria, giving as one of the reasons that eradication has been a success in Venezuela in spite of the presence of lots of monkeys (10). This shows a considerable degree of unbiologic thinking, for the monkeys of Venezuela are much different from those of Asia. It is not permissible to use the experience there and apply it directly to Africa and Malaya without some modifications. At the time of writing (September 1962), no monkey malaria from America has ever been transmitted successfully to man by a mosquito under controlled laboratory conditions. To understand the position, a brief discussion on the origins of man and monkey in America is necessary.

There are theoretical reasons for believing, first, that primate malaria of America should differ from that of the Old World, and secondly, that human malaria is a recently introduced infection, imported only since the time of Columbus. An imported infection is more susceptible to eradication procedures than one native to the country which has deep evolutionary and ecologic roots there.

America has been separated geographically from the rest of the world for a very long time. There are theories or guesses that it once was part of the rest but drifted away, as in Wegener's theory of continental drift, or that a land bridge once connected it with Africa or Australia. Even if one of these did prove to be correct, the separation must have happened long before the primates appeared on earth, so that there has been no way for the monkeys on the one land mass to come into contact with those on the other. To quote Romer: "Little is known of the fossil history of the American monkeys, although there are some remains from the middle to late Cenozoic beds in South America. They are as advanced as Old World monkeys in certain regards, more primitive in others. At first sight, one would tend to say that they form an intermediate stage in the evolution of monkeys from lower primates. But the facts of geography are against this. Quite surely they never lived anywhere but in South America, separated by a broad ocean from the Old World, where the evolution of higher monkeys and apes began at an early time. There are no fossil remains of monkeys of any sort in

North America. Hence it is probable that monkeys evolved from high *Tarsius*—like lemuroids twice, in parallel fashion—once in South America; once, more successfully in Eurasia and Africa" (11).

If this is the case, then there is no reason to expect that the parasites of the one set of monkeys should be closely related to those of the other; to the contrary, one would suppose them to have substantial differences. Of course, should the American monkeys have become infected with human malaria in the past few hundred years, as is believed to have happened in the case of yellow fever (12), then the story would be vastly different and eradication is going to be very difficult.

Man is the only primate to colonize successfully the Americas from the Old World, and most certainly he first came via the Bering land bridge. It has been mentioned earlier that during the Ice Age America was joined to Asia by land, since the frozen water lowered the sea level by some hundreds of feet. The Bering straits are only a little over a hundred feet deep today, while 20,000 years ago they were above sea level. Furthermore, at that time the ice sheets did not cover all this land, so that there was a straight passage for both man and animal migrants from one continent to another. In spite of the proximity of the ice, the climate would have been a little warmer perhaps than today, since the cold water of the Arctic Ocean would have no access to the Pacific, which would therefore have a higher temperature in the northern region than at present.

The man of Asia 20,000 years ago, of course, would not have known of the land waiting for him in America. He would be engaged in hunting and would follow the migrating herds of mammoth and musk ox and caribou. These would lead him across to Alaska, where his spear points have been found in the soil, mingled with the bones of the extinct elephant, bison, camel, horse, and an extinct jaguar called the Alaskan lion (13). From there, his most promising routes would have been along the valley of the Yukon to the Mackenzie valley and then south along the east side of the Rockies. During the last glaciation, the Wisconsin, about 40,000 years ago, the ice retreated, leaving a corridor from north to south in this area; then about 15,000 years ago all the ice receded and left the whole area clear. The melting of the ice raised the sea level and broke off the land bridge, so that people arriving after perhaps 10,000 years ago would have to come from Asia either across the ice or by boat. A full listing of all finds of ancient man in North America to 1957 has been compiled by Wormington (14).

The peoples that would make the trip from Asia would belong to any wandering group that happened to be in the right spot. These would be a mixed stock of people and not confined merely to Mongoloid types, but whatever their stock, they would be unlikely to be infected with malaria in their northern Asian homeland. Even if they had malaria in Siberia or eastern Asia, they would have lost it long before they reached those parts of the New World warm enough to permit mosquito transmission of the plasmodium. The travels in the Arctic and sub-Arctic must have taken hundreds or even thousands of years. It is, therefore, suggested that the original inhabitants of the New World were free of malaria when they arrived, and that the infection was only introduced in very recent times. In comparison with the Old World, it should, therefore, be fairly easy to eradicate it, unless the monkeys have already become infected with the human strain.

What, therefore, is the future of malaria eradication? In my opinion it will go smoothly and quickly where there are no monkeys and in areas like America where it has probably been recently introduced (Figure 15). It will go more slowly in certain underdeveloped countries, and not at all in places with fighting and civil unrest. In general, progress will be made until the disease is no longer a public health problem on a world scale. However, in many places with large numbers of monkeys infected with forms of plasmodium that are easily transmissible to man by the prevailing species of mosquitoes, eradication as defined here will not be possible by present techniques. The best to be achieved is likely to be a state in which the human population is cleared of infection, but where occasional spread occurs from monkeys, further passage can occur by mosquitoes from man to man, and at least some of the potential mosquito vectors will feed on either man or monkey. If the evolution of malaria as propounded in this book is anywhere near the truth, then the spread of plasmodia from one type of host to the other—either from monkey to man, or the reverse—is most likely as at least an occasional event. Let us suppose it happens in only one case of malaria in ten thousand. In a control program, this amount of infection would be completely insignificant and indeed very difficult to demonstrate. But in the final stages of an eradication program, it would become the dominant feature. In the first place, normally there would probably be competition in nature between the human and primate types, with the former being the fitter for humans: with the human parasites out of the way, the primate ones would have a clear field for ex-

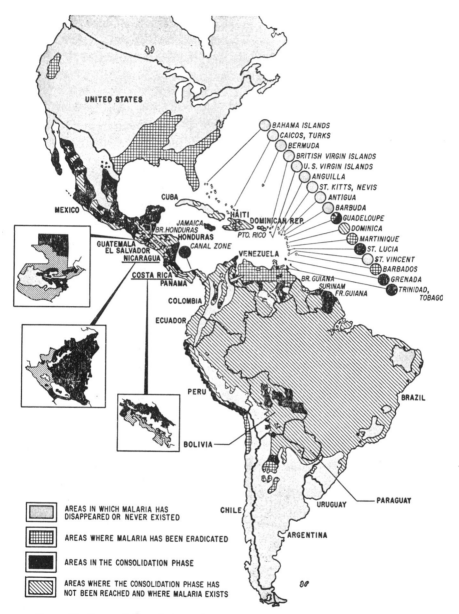

Figure 15. Status of the malaria eradication program in the Americas, August 1, 1962. (Courtesy of Pan American Health Organization)

pansion to the human population. Once the eradication program had been completed and the whole organization dismantled, this one case in ten thousand could become all important as a source of re-infection of the area.

The position will then be like that of yellow fever in South America in which the human population can be protected from all except the occasional case from the forest regions. This, of course, is a very desirable state to reach, but will mean the provision of surveillance teams for an indefinite period of time in the future, and preparations for occasional outbreaks of disease.*

POLIOMYELITIS

Evolution

Poliomyelitis is obviously an ancient disease, for there is an excellent engraving on stone of a man with the residual paralysis from Egypt (Plate II). Yet it was so rare that it was not recognized as a clinical entity until about two centuries ago.

When first discovered, it was primarily an affliction of children. Heine described the clinical aspects in some detail in the years 1838–60 and named the disease "Spinal Infantile Paralysis." In the past half century, the picture has changed and increasingly the main brunt is falling on the adults. The recognition that the essential lesion was in the spinal cord was made by Laborde in 1864. In 1908, Landsteiner transmitted the disease to a monkey. Within a few years, the agent had been recovered from the stools of patients, but the significance of this observation was not appreciated for some decades (15).

It is customary to attribute the increasing commonness of the infection in the more developed countries, as well as the greater involvement of the adult population, to improvements in hygiene. The argument is that prevention of the spread of intestinal pathogens hinders infection of the young infant while still protected by its

* As the book goes to press July 18 to July 26, 1963, it is understood that a South American primate *Plasmodium* has been successfully transmitted to man. Apparently, Dr. P. G. Contacos and his workers at the State Penitentiary, Atlanta, Georgia, have passaged *P. braziliensis* to human volunteers by both syringe and mosquito. This work may have great significance for the malaria eradication program in South America. To what extent the program will be effected will not be known until considerable field studies have been carried out.

mother's antibodies. Instead, infection takes place in later life when the individual is highly susceptible. In underdeveloped countries, where the chances of infection with any of the locally prevailing organisms are so great that infants must acquire them soon after birth, poliomyelitis is a rare disease. Significantly, there have been two sharp epidemics in Japan and Ceylon in the past year: both of these countries are in the vanguard of Asian countries so far as hygiene is concerned. Colombo in Ceylon had one of the best water supplies in Asia until overgrowth of the population strained its capacity.

Eradication

Great efforts have been made in recent times to prepare an adequate vaccine against poliomyelitis, particularly in the United States. The problem has proved very difficult, in spite of the epoch-making advances in growing viruses in tissue culture made by Enders and his group of workers. Several times complete success has seemed to be achieved, but only at the last minute has disaster occurred or incomplete success been the reward. By the present time, the main contenders for acceptance are the vaccines of Salk and Sabin. The former is a killed vaccine given by injection and the latter an attenuated live one given orally. So far as eradication is concerned, the former will not be discussed here, for while it provides considerable protection by stimulating adequate quantities of antibodies in the blood, it does not prevent growth of the virus in the intestine. Consequently, while it often inhibits the appearance of the disease, it does not stop the immunized individual from carrying the virus (Figure 16).

The Sabin vaccine seems to give solid immunity both to the individual and also to the community, if a high enough percentage of the population is protected. Cincinnati was the first large city in the U.S. to have mass immunization. In 1960, Dr. Albert B. Sabin gave the city and surrounding Hamilton County enough vaccine made by himself to immunize on an experimental basis all of those 18 years of age and under. The vaccine was distributed by volunteers and almost 80 per cent of the age groups offered it were immunized (16). Dr. Sabin kept a surveillance for the disease in 1960 and found only one case, this being a person who obviously had been infected outside of the city and county (17). In 1961, further offers of the vaccine were made to the children and babies of the city, and the level of immunity was maintained. I maintained the surveillance in

1961 and again no indigenous case of the disease could be found (18). In 1962, the vaccine was licensed and became commercially available on the market, and large quantities were being used both by the city and volunteer agencies and private physicians, when in June the first possible case of poliomyelitis was diagnosed that could possibly have been infected in the city. The baby had Type III in-

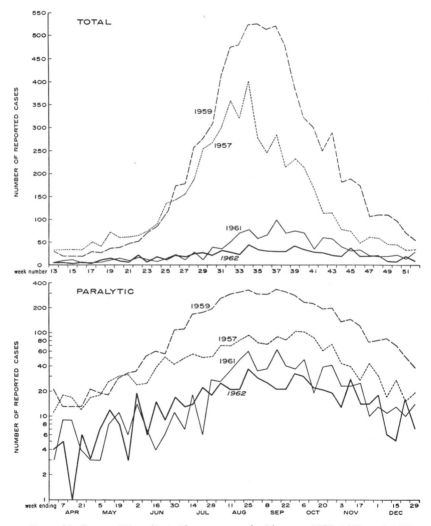

Figure 16. Current U.S. polio incidence compared with years 1957, 1959, and 1961, April–December, by week. (Data provided by the National Office of Vital Statistics and Communicable Disease Center, U.S. Public Health Service, Atlanta, Ga.)

fection. It had been taken by its mother outside of the city on three occasions during the period ten days to three weeks before onset of the disease. It had also been in contact with a child that had received Type III vaccine. Whether the baby was infected inside or outside the city or as a result of contact with the Type III vaccine has been hotly debated and no conclusion reached. I personally do not think it was naturally infected within the city limits, and if so, then there has been no case of poliomyelitis in Cincinnati for three years. This experience of Cincinnati is the best evidence we have in the U.S. that a sizable population—half a million people in the city and as many more in the county and neighboring areas—can in fact be protected in this fashion.

Unfortunately, a number of cases of poliomyelitis have been found in persons given Type III vaccine, and this has indicated some doubt as to its effectiveness. At the time of writing (October 1962) contradictory statements are being issued almost daily by opposing authorities. It seems clear, however, that the risk of coming down with poliomyelitis after taking the vaccine is a very small one. Eleven cases so far have been reported in association with Type III. Even if all of these were caused by the vaccine, which is by no means clearly proved, the risk is only about one in a million, which makes the vaccine much safer than penicillin and very much safer than smallpox vaccination. The only possible case of disease occurring by contact with a vaccinated person is the one described above in Cincinnati, and it is a doubtful one.

The main characteristic of the Sabin vaccine that makes it so strong a candidate in the race to eradicate poliomyelitis—in addition to its capacity to give solid immunity—is its ease of administration and the high level of public acceptance. The dose of two or three drops can be given on a spoon or lump of sugar. No elaborate system of sterilizing thousands of syringes is needed and the whole operation can be carried out with non-medical volunteers with only the minimum of medical supervision. This can be illustrated by Cincinnati's experience. Following the diagnosis in 1962 of the case of Type III infection described above, Cincinnati and the five counties in the surrounding area organized a mass campaign to immunize that section of the population that had not been given the vaccine two years earlier. The speed with which this was done is instructive. The disease was first diagnosed clinically on Monday as being poliomyelitis, and the virus was isolated and identified as Type III by Saturday morning. That afternoon, a conference was held between the Health Department, the Academy of Medicine, and Dr. Sabin, when it was agreed that a mass campaign for the city was needed. An emergency meeting of the Academy was held next day on Sunday morning, when the Academy decided to sponsor a program not only for the city but also the county, and that the vaccine should be given the following Sunday. Soon all five counties agreed to join. It seemed to some that seven days was not time enough to launch such an ambitious program successfully, but the people rose to the occasion. With saturation publicity, volunteer workers came forward in masses, and in three days the city alone had 50 centers set up in schools, each staffed with 30 volunteers, a physician, pharmacist, nurse, school principal, bank teller to collect contributions to pay for the vaccine, firemen to control traffic, and boy scouts to guide people. The five counties had similar organizations. When the seventh day came, all went smoothly, and more than 700,000 people were given the vaccine. A clinic of the type described could have served 15 or 20,000 people in six hours had it been necessary. There was no waiting, the movement in and out of the clinic being steady as shown in the photographs. The only time queues formed was when temporary shortages of vaccine occurred (Plates IX to XII).

With the vaccine so easy to give, the mass immunization of a country becomes highly practical, and indeed many nations outside of the U.S.A. have already achieved this. In Russia, many tens of millions have been immunized and also populations in several countries of Europe. Czechoslovakia immunized its people in 1960, and since that time there has been no polio in the country. On a country-wide scale, this is excellent, but what of the world as a whole? There the prospect is not so promising. As mentioned above, the emerging countries have very little clinical disease, but the virus is obviously present. In my travels in Africa and Asia over a period of seven years, I saw only two cases in Colombo and heard of another in Chittagong in East Pakistan, these being in peoples native to those areas. On the other hand, there were three cases among the very small western population in East Pakistan in 1959, and a very sharp outbreak among the Americans in Karachi in 1956–57. In Karachi, 17 Americans out of a total population of about 600 or 700 developed paralysis of varying degrees, an exceedingly high attack rate.

In an emerging country, it is difficult enough selling to the government the idea of spending money on any health matter, but it would be almost impossible to try and put over a program for a disease which the government has heard of only in the foreign newspapers. It would be far more difficult than trying to sell the U.S.A. on the eradication of *Aedes aegypti*. It may be that in time, as the hygienic conditions improve and polio begins to emerge, as has happened in Japan and Ceylon in the past year, that the position will change markedly, but at the moment, the eradication of polio on a world scale scarcely seems practical.

Even if it were eradicated, there is a serious danger that other agents might evolve to take its place. There are lots of enteroviruses capable of attacking the nervous system, and in particular the Coxackie group. One of these can even now cause paralysis like polio and so has been called Type 4 poliovirus by the Russians. Obviously, a tight system of surveillance is essential, long after the last indication of active infection with the polioviruses has disappeared from a community.

Production of live attenuated virus for use as an immunizing agent gives some hope that, through oral vaccination of large numbers of individuals, the wild virulent strains will be replaced by harmless strains. What is being suggested is a practical test of a bitterly fought theoretical problem, known to biologists as Gause's principle or the "competitive exclusion" principle of Hardin (19). In its simplest form this can be stated as follows: "Two related species of the same ecology cannot live together in the same place," for one species will have an advantage over the other and in time will replace it. The question in poliomyelitis will be, which species will survive, the virulent wild virus or the vaccine? If it is proposed merely to release doses of the vaccine in the hope that it will spread under its own agency and replace the other virus, then the effort is almost certainly doomed to failure, for the wild strains have been selected under intensely competitive conditions over long periods and presumably are far better adapted to life under natural conditions than is any "hothouse" laboratory strain that is liberated. The all-important capacity to resist adverse circumstances while being transmitted from host to host in nature has been ignored during the passage procedures in the laboratory, for passive transfer by syringe or pipet is not likely to have encouraged the selection of strains resistant to adverse conditions outside the body. As a result, the vaccine virus can be expected to have relatively little capacity to move to new hosts, as compared with the wild strains, and is unlikely to become established as a self-perpetuating organism. The experience of the Russians has shown that about 50 per cent of the contacts of protected persons excrete live vaccine within three to five months after vaccination (20), but in contrast it is well known that during epidemics of the wild strains, almost everyone in a small, intimate community is infected. Experience in the United States indicates that the vaccine virus spreads poorly and does not establish itself as a permanent infection (21). The differences in spread in the U.S.S.R. and in the United States may be related to variations in sanitary conditions.

Elsewhere it has been proposed that for every infection and set of circumstances there is a minimum host population that is necessary to support the infection on a permanent endemic basis (Chapter 4). The fact that poliomyelitis infection dies out in small communities has been recognized (22). In a large human population, the number of individuals susceptible to the virulent poliomyelitis infection can be reduced below this threshold level by repeated feedings of the competing attenuated and immunizing live virus. When this threshold is passed, the virulent wild virus will automatically die out. The percentage of susceptible individuals in the community that form this threshold population will vary from one population to another, being lower where the chance of person-to-person contact is high, as in areas with, say, 1,000 persons per square mile, and high in areas with only five or ten persons per square mile. To state this another way, it may be necessary to immunize 90 per cent of the people in a town and only 75 per cent in a rural area to reach the threshold level at which the wild virus disappears.

In eradication programs confined to a continent, there will be no means of keeping out reinfecting imported strains, for there is no practical way of detecting carriers of poliovirus. This means that occasional cases of poliomyelitis will occur, but that, at the worst, any epidemic resulting will be small and sharply limited. It does not follow that, if the whole world were brought up to the required level of immunity and the wild strains of virulent virus became extinct, these strains would have been eradicated for good and all further efforts could be abandoned. The circumstances that led to the evolution of the wild strains will presumably still be operative, and natural selection would quickly produce new strains from the vaccine virus, or related enteroviruses so that the immunizing procedures would have to be maintained indefinitely. By practical definition, this situation would be one of control and not eradication.

TUBERCULOSIS

Evolution

The outstanding characteristic of the genus *Mycobacterium* is its possession in its coverings of a lipoidal material that makes bacilli acid-fast to certain stains. Not all the members of the genus always have this acid-fast quality and there are members of other genera that can also be acid-fast, but by and large this is the outstanding feature of its various species. This material is of considerable importance in the protection of the organism both from adverse physical conditions as well as the defenses of the host in which it is living, so that its possession is a matter of considerable survival importance to an organism. Bergey's *Manual of Determinative Bacteriology* lists thirteen species of *Mycobacteria,* including those causing disease in mammals, birds, reptiles, fish, and others apparently being commensals; still others are thought to be free living in soil. With such a wide range of environments colonized by the organisms, there are two main possibilities as to their origins; either all species of *Mycobacterium* are descended from a common ancestor dating back to very ancient times, or else the lipoidal material has been evolved independently on a number of occasions by differing organisms. In the latter case, a superficial resemblance due to its possession would be resulting from convergent evolution and has resulted in unrelated species being wrongly placed in the genus *Mycobacterium.* Which of these two possibilities are correct cannot be known at this time, but since bacteriologists seldom seem to question that all the species do indeed belong to the one genus, the assumption will be made here that they were in fact derived from one common ancestor.

This being the case, then the extent of the distribution of mycobacteria as free-living organisms, commensals, and parasites in a wide range of habitats including soil, warm-blooded mammals and birds, cold-blooded reptiles and lizards, and fishes living in both fresh and salt water indicates that this genus must have been in existence many hundreds of millions of years. Of course, it is possible that it evolved much more recently and spread rapidly to all these places in more modern times, but the range of distribution is so great that it scarcely seems likely. The association with animals must have begun at a time when all creatures lived in the sea; as the land was invaded first by the mud-crawling fishes and amphibians, the acid-fast organisms living in them would go also. As time passed and the reptiles appeared, these in turn giving rise to the birds and mammals, the organisms would speciate in parallel with their hosts. During the long eras that have passed, a considerable degree of adaptation would have occurred between hosts and parasites so that in general, lines of organisms would have developed that were so specialized that they could live in no other hosts than their chosen ones. This has been called "vertical" transmission in Chapter 3. In man, the representative of this type would be *M. leprae* which has not been grown with any great success in any animal apart from man, and in cattle it would be the agent of Johne's disease.

At the same time, from the beginning there would have been organisms which, from the nature of things, would become more widely distributed and, therefore, not allowed to become so highly specialized. Bird parasites, for example, can be carried over vast distances, the droppings are scattered indiscriminately, while birds themselves are liable to be eaten by predators of all kinds, including mammals, reptiles and fish. Bird mycobacteria are, therefore, widely distributed. This is "horizontal" transmission, but in time, repeated transmission within a new host would produce a new strain of the parasite. It is suggested here that horizontal spread of this kind produced the *Mycobacteria* that caused tuberculosis in man and his domestic cattle, once man had settled down with his agriculture and domesticated animals. As described earlier in this book, sometime between 6000–8000 B.C., man learned to grow crops and to tame and use animals. This had many significant results, including bringing him into contact of a very intimate nature with these animals. The animals themselves would, of course, experience a considerable change from life in the wild, including confinement in sheds during the winter, changes of diet, the cessation of constant migration in search of food and water, and closer contact with other cattle.

Now wild animals do not commonly have tuberculosis in the natural state, although it does occur. My experience while in charge of the animals in the Regents Park Menagerie, London, is that most of the tuberculosis seen under such conditions develops after the confinement of the animal.

Once I had one bittern brought in sick, having been found in the streets of London. When it died a few days later, an autopsy showed advanced tuberculosis.

I have dissected many wild animals, birds, and snakes after I had shot or trapped them while in West Africa, and none had tuberculosis. However, a squacco heron that was reared as a pet died of the disease after about ten months (23). In 1948, through the assistance of Dr. Archer of the Lamont Clinic, Alberta, I was able to watch the tuberculin testing of 400 American Buffalo (bison) in Elk Island National Park, Alberta. These buffalo live under natural conditions in this large park and all were tuberculin negative; a much larger herd than this at Wainwright, some distance away, proved to be heavily infected, but this one shared the range with domestic cattle. A wild animal suffering from tuberculosis of an acute nature would not survive long in the fierce competition in nature. Also a nomadic herbivore living in the outdoors has only a small chance of acquiring the infection from another animal; it is, therefore, suggested here that the modern type of acute infection developed only since the domestication of animals, when transmission became easy because man fed and cared for them.

For much the same reasons, man must also have developed tuberculosis because the development of agriculture made him live a sedentary life, in ever-increasing numbers in crowded towns. Tuberculosis is not basically a disease of the rural areas, although it can have disastrous effects when it spreads there from the urban regions. Even less is it a disease of the nomad with a hunting economy. In an earlier chapter the account has been given of the disastrous epidemic that broke out in the Indians of Saskatchewan after they had been settled on the land. Prior to that time, tuberculosis had been a rare disease among them. It has been much the same story for all small isolated groups all over the world, whether it was the African in South Africa, the Maori in New Zealand, the Polynesian in the Pacific, or the Aborigine in Australia. Furthermore, the clinical form of the disease in such peoples differs from that seen in urban dwellers, being more acute in nature and characterized more by glandular involvement than pulmonary cavitation (see Chapter 4). The general impression exists that even among the more densely populated countries there exist gradations in the susceptibility to the disease, with the Jews at one end of the scale being highly resistant and the Irish at the other being very susceptible. The usual explanation given is that the Jewish people have been living for centuries in crowded ghettos, while the Irish have been largely farmers in a sparsely populated land. The conclusion must be drawn that the infection is one of the crowd diseases, discussed under Theories 4 and 5, and could not have existed in its present form before the creation of towns and urban life, and therefore must have appeared after the development of agriculture made possible the foundations of such cultures.

An interesting suggestion made in recent years is that the predominant acid-fast infection existing 2,000 years ago in Europe was leprosy, but that this gave way as the new infection of tuberculosis invaded the continent. The basis for this suggestion is that, first, leprosy apparently did die out in the Middle Ages in Europe, to survive only in parts of Scandinavia, and secondly, that the leprosy and tuberculosis organisms seem to give a certain degree of cross-immunity against one another. Neither of these points can be claimed as facts. The diagnosis of leprosy from descriptions that have survived a thousand years is a very difficult matter, and there is little certainty that the diseases were in fact what is known as Hansens disease today. Just because churches in England sometimes have leper windows and there were leper houses in various locations does not indicate that the condition was caused by *M. leprae*. However, it still undoubtedly persisted in Norway, and recent studies in Denmark, which now is free of the disease, show that skeletons in churchyards dating back many hundreds of years do have bone lesions of leprosy (24). These are found in areas where the disease has not been seen in modern times. It is, therefore, possible that leprosy did occur in areas of Europe that have been clear of it for centuries.

The cross-immunity between the organisms of the two diseases is difficult to demonstrate, since efforts to grow the *M. leprae* on medium or in animals have been very unrewarding. However, complement-fixing antibodies against antigens from tubercle bacilli can be demonstrated easily in sera from leprous cases (25).* Much evidence has come from Brazil and Japan, and consists of tests with lepromin and tuberculin in people with leprosy. Lepromin is a preparation made from human leprosy tissue which contains swarms of the leprosy bacilli. There does seem to be some degree of positivity of the skin tests using such preparations on individuals suffering from the opposite infections, but the evidence is by no means clear-cut.

---

* McFadzean (25a) has reported the following:
1. Forty-eight patients with leprosy were injected intradermally with lepromin, tuberculin, and antigens prepared from B.C.G., *M. fortuitum, M. rhodocrous, M. marinum, M. phlei,* and *M. smegmatis.*
2. There was no correlation between the reactions to lepromin and the reactions to any other antigens.
3. The reactions to tuberculin were significantly correlated with the reactions to *M. marinum* both at 72 hours and when the reactions at 72 hours to tuberculin were compared with the reactions at 21 days to *M. marinum.*

The best experiment so far carried out—and it is by no means above criticism—is some Japanese work in which children of leprous parents were immunized with BCG and watched to see if they developed leprosy. There were 248 in the experiment, with one set of children kept as controls and not given BCG vaccination. The morbidity was high in the control group without the BCG vaccination, so that the conclusion was drawn that such a vaccination did give a good measure of protection. The protection seemed to be of value even after infection had apparently occurred (26).

If it is accepted that leprosy at one time was common in Europe and that there is a considerable degree of cross-immunity between leprosy and tuberculosis infections, then it does seem possible that the former was replaced by the latter during the Middle Ages. It would be in conformity with Theory 4 as expressed in Chapter 4, in which in a large population a rapidly spreading infection would replace a chronic, slowly transmitted one. Tuberculosis would be an acute infection at first. In a susceptible population lacking any high degree of genetic resistance, it is much more of a rapidly progressing infection than that seen today in Western peoples living in urban areas. When it first appeared in Europe, it probably would be much more like the rapidly advancing glandular type seen today in Africans, the Maori, and other such recently infected people as described above.

Theory 3 states that populations tend to become genetically resistant to the pathogens to which they are exposed, so that some such resistance to tuberculosis could be expected to have developed in those people suffering from it over the centuries. Indeed, the Saskatchewan Indians seem to be acquiring this over a few generations as described in Chapter 4. However, there are so many factors operating in a disease like tuberculosis that the influence of any single one is almost impossible to measure with any accuracy, especially since experiments with humans are very difficult to perform. Still, there do seem to be racial differences among Western peoples as mentioned above, with the Jews at one extreme being fairly resistant to the disease and the Irish at the other extreme being unduly susceptible.

Eradication

Tuberculosis has now displaced malaria as the world's number one problem in infectious diseases. It is found in all countries of the world and is the cause of appalling sickness and death in many areas. In the past half century, its occurrence in the Western civilizations has shown a marked tendency downwards, so that by the 1930's many people were encouraged to anticipate the complete disappearance of the disease without any more control measures being needed than were already being applied. Frost asked the question as to how much control was needed to obtain this result and speculated that the infection would die out of its own accord if the conditions of his time continued (27). During and after World War II, a series of dramatic discoveries in the field of chemotherapy, including the discoveries of

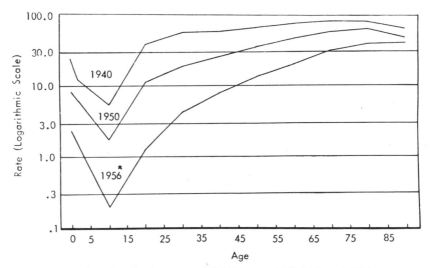

Figure 17. Tuberculosis death rates per 100,000 by age 1940, 1950, and 1956

This chart shows the tremendous variation with age in tuberculosis death rates. For 1956 the rate among preschool children (1.6) was 8 times the rate among school-age children (0.2). The rate among persons over age 65 (34.3) was 26 times the rate for young adults aged 15 to 24 (1.3).

The logarithmic scale presentation permits the observation that the improvement in death rates has been greater for young people than for older people, and also that the change from 1950 to 1956 exceeds the change from 1940 to 1950, for all age groups.

During the first quarter of this century, death rates were greatest among young adults, especially in the age group 25 to 34. The curve for 1940 shows only a vestige of the hump that used to exist, and by 1950 the hump was gone, for the nation as a whole. Later charts show that the young adult hump was still present in 1956 to some degree for portions of our population. (The symbol "1956" is used as a shorthand notation for the average of data for 1955, 1956, and 1957. The average was used to produce more stable data for statistical analysis.)

Source: The Arden House Conference on Tuberculosis, 1959. U.S. Department of Health, Education, and Welfare, P.H.S. Publication No. 784, Washington, D.C. Data supplied through the courtesy of the Communicable Disease Center, U.S. Public Health Service, Atlanta, Ga.

streptomycin and isoniazid have advanced greatly the hopes in this direction (Figures 17, 18), so that at the conference at Arden House (28) in 1959, the following recommendations were made:

The major recommendation of the conference is a program for the widespread application of chemotherapy as a public health measure for the elimination of tuberculosis in the United States:

> *GOAL:* To sterilize that important part of the reservoir of tubercle bacilli that presently exists throughout the country in persons currently suffering from active tuberculous disease, whether presently known or unknown to public health authorities, and in selected persons who previously have had active disease and were inadequately treated.
>
> *TECHNIQUE:* Mobilize all resources for a widespread application of the scientifically demonstrated and medically accepted procedures of adequate chemotherapy. These include

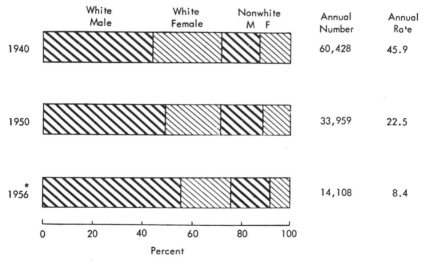

Figure 18. Race-sex distribution of Tuberculosis deaths, 1940, 1950, and 1956.

This chart shows the progressive concentration of tuberculosis deaths among white males so that, by 1956, 55 per cent of the tuberculosis deaths were in this one group. This has occurred primarily because rates for white females have improved faster than rates for white males; also because rates for non-whites have improved faster than rates for whites.

While non-whites still have death rates nearly three times as high as the death rates for whites, only a quarter of the deaths are among non-whites. (The symbol "1956" is used as a shorthand notation for the average of data for 1955, 1956, and 1957. The average was used to produce more stable data for statistical analysis.)

Source: The Arden House Conference on Tuberculosis, 1959. Data supplied through the courtesy of the Communicable Disease Center, U.S. Public Health Service, Atlanta, Ga.

the proper dosage of appropriate drugs or combination of drugs given continuously over an adequate period of time—procedures that are known to destroy tubercle bacilli in the human body, render the patient's disease non-communicable to others, and minimize the possibility of reactivation.

The unique aspect of this recommendation lies in its emphasis on such chemotherapy primarily as a public health tuberculosis control measure (as well as for the benefit of the individual patient), with all of the connotations of community mobilization and control by public health authorities that this new concept implies. This recommendation obviously implies as well an adequate case detection program.

Unfortunately, the definition of eradication often used at the conference was not that given in this book. The term most used was "eradication as a public health problem" and to me such a phrase is meaningless and even a self-contradiction. However, this concept is the one that seems to be generally held by workers in the field of tuberculosis, and the ideas expressed in this book are not acceptable to many of them. There was a seminar on Tuberculosis Eradication at the annual American Public Health Association meeting at Detroit in 1961, where Dr. Fred L. Soper, whose concept is that of "pulling out by the roots," was the invited speaker. The seminar showed clearly that many tuberculosis workers did not like this concept.

The opportunity to test the possibility of eradicating tuberculosis down to the last single case arose in 1961 with my appointment as Assistant Commissioner of Health of Cincinnati. In this capacity, I found myself being, among other matters, in charge of the tuberculosis program for a city of some half million people. In the previous two years, the people of the city had been sensitized to the idea of mass health research programs through the campaigns to test the vaccines against poliomyelitis using the Sabin and Salk vaccines. In 1961, a Health Department Study Group on Tuberculosis was set up which included most of the experts on that disease in the city and, after some six month deliberation, it was agreed unanimously that complete eradication was both desirable and possible in Cincinnati. An announcement to that effect was made early in 1962, with the 15-year program to commence on September 1, 1962 (Table 17). On September 9, 1962, a Seminar on Tuberculosis Eradication for Practitioners was held in the Academy of Medicine and about 150 attended, representing more than 10 per cent of all physicians in the city and the area around. Most of the interested voluntary agencies and the Board of Education are collaborating in the effort. Cincinnati is thus the first city in the world to proclaim openly that it intends to wipe out tuberculosis down to the last single indigenous case and thus eradicate the disease. In assessing the degree of success in this operation, any cases found in the city due to importation of the infection from outside will not be considered as indigenous infections.

Having defined what is meant by eradication, the next step is to do the same for the disease itself. In Cincinnati, we are trying to wipe out only the organism *M. tuberculosis* and not all the forms of

TABLE 17. TUBERCULOSIS ERADICATION IN CINCINNATI

	A Suggested Timetable by T. Aidan Cockburn, M.D., D.P.H.
Before September 1, 1962	Planning
Year 1 (Sept. '62–'63)	Preparing for eradication: Testing techniques Training of staff Intensifying control measures Tuberculin testing (one grade) Preventive Isoniazid therapy.
Years 2–5 ('63–'67)	Eradication proceeding, with progressive tightening of procedures, until maximum efforts being achieved.
Years 6–10 ('68–'72)	Complete cessation of transmission in Cincinnati except for introduced infection.
Year 11 ('73)	All children arriving in school tuberculin negative and staying in that state.

This is based upon the efforts of the City alone, without outside assistance. With about $50,000.00 per annum outside aid, the process could be shortened by one or more years.

disease caused by the various acid-fast bacilli belonging to other species of the genus *Mycobacterium*. This means that if the effort is successful, there would still be occurring disease due to the other members of the genus. *M. bovis* is not a problem, since there are not many milk cows in the city area and all of these have been tuberculin tested. All milk is pasteurized and a close check is maintained by the city sanitarians of all milk-processing plants and farms supplying milk to the city. On a national scale, the eradication of bovine tuberculosis has been pursued for many years by the Department of Agriculture with a considerable degree of success, but as mentioned earlier, eradication in its strictest sense has not been reached since the disease still exists among the cattle (29).

There are a number of other acid-fast bacilli, called variously the atypical or anonymous organisms, that can be found in association with pathological lesions in both cattle and humans. At present these are classified into four groups according to the conditions under which they do or do not produce pigment in culture. Some of these are clearly parasites of birds, while some may or may not be free-living organisms capable of causing disease when infecting mammals. Much research will be necessary before the status of such organisms is defined but one thing is certain, that they will be largely unaffected by any campaign to eradicate human tuberculosis. The birds and other environments that form their main reservoirs will be outside the scope of any campaign that Cincinnati or any other city or area is likely to undertake within the foreseeable future. Much the same goes for the *Mycobacterium* spread by water, at first called *M. balnei,* but now regarded to be the same as the fish pathogen *M. marinum.* The eradication program in Cincinnati will, therefore, be aimed basically at the extinction of *M. tuberculosis,* the human pathogen.

In a program of this kind, the only important type of case to be considered is the infectious one capable of infecting other people. Non-infectious cases are important only to the degree to which they might become infectious again. The first important task is, therefore, to regard every infectious case of tuberculosis as an acute public health emergency. There are two kinds of such cases, those that are known and those that are not. In Cincinnati, at the time of writing, are 279 known acute cases of tuberculosis (Table 17), and I have them all listed on a peg board, with colored pegs next to their numbers giving such important details as the stage of follow-up of their contacts, whether hospitalized or not, their sputum status, and the degree of sensitivity of their organisms to chemotherapy. This peg board is revised daily, and any patient not isolated properly or not under threatment is "red flagged" until brought under control. The next task is to find the infectious cases that are not yet known and add them to the list on the peg board. The routine ways of doing this are, of course, the diagnoses by physicians in practice, routine radiograms of foodhandlers, teachers, etc., and the search for cases among contacts. In addition, there is the search for sources of infection of school children found to be tuberculin positive at school. To these can be added special programs for the screening either by radiogram or tuberculin test of all persons of all ages except the very young, living in areas of especially high incidence. When the 279 acute cases of tuberculosis were pinned on a map, it was immediately evident that 60 per cent of them were located in two comparatively small areas. These areas have a combined population of 120,000 people, mostly Negro, and this number is within the resources of the city so far as mass screening is concerned. The Anti-Tuberculosis League normally x-rays 60,000 people in a year. Only those above the age of 18 will be x-rayed, the children being skin tested in school. Such a mass screening of one of the two areas had been carried out in 1950 and the results had been very disappointing in that few cases of tuberculosis had been found. What probably happened was that the people with the disease did not go to be x-rayed, so that next time an effort must be made to make certain that everyone in the area comes for examination.

The people next in importance to those with active disease are those who have been infected and who may develop active lesions sometime in the future. These are the quiescent and inactive cases and those with large skin reactions to tuberculin or those who are recent converters. These need careful watching and perhaps preventive chemotherapy. In Cincinnati, all children that are recent converters, or have reactions more than 15 mms. in diameter, or are skin-test positive contacts of cases will be offered isoniazid prophylactically.

In a large American city today, there is no reason why any person diagnosed as having active tuberculosis should not be isolated efficiently in some fashion and commence proper treatment within a week. With modern chemotherapy, the great majority of cases cease to be infective within quite a short time, and to those that do not respond in this fashion, there are available a wide range of medical and surgical measures that are very effective. There are some people who have economic or psychological handicaps that make them try to abandon their treatments before they are considered to be noninfective. For these there are the assistances provided by the Welfare Departments or the voluntary organizations; in the last resort the courts will usually authorize compulsion if necessary. Of our 279 cases probably only a handful—say 20 or 25—will be difficult to handle. After they have been dealt with, will come the task of constant screening for undiscovered cases and prophylactic chemotherapy for prevention of disease in those already infected.

In all matters like this, a means of measurement of success is needed to estimate the effectiveness of the program as it continues. We have chosen the children entering school as our indicator, and the percentages of these that are skin-test positive when first tested will be our measurements of success. In six years time we hope to see a marked reduction in this percentage, and total success will be achieved when all those children native to the city, admitted to school for the first time, are found to be tuberculin negative and stay that way during their school life.

While we can thus plan for a small area like Cincinnati, it is otherwise for vast countries like India or Indonesia where tuberculosis is very common and the resources are few. For such places eradication is not to be considered at the present, and even control is a doubtful matter. The answer there lies more in immunization with BCG vaccination as described in the last chapter on Ceylon, rather than building hospitals or treating patients in their homes with drugs like isoniazid. Eradication on a world scale must be only a dream for a long time to come.

A potent tool in tuberculosis is vaccination with BCG. There is little or no doubt that this immunizing agent provides a very substantial protection against tuberculosis, lasting many years, and its use is the method of choice in areas of high incidence. However, in Cincinnati, our chief tool is the tuberculin test and this would be seriously damaged by any city-wide BCG program. As the cases of active disease diminish toward the zero mark, this disadvantage of BCG vaccine begins to outweigh its advantages, so that there is little room for it in our operation. Quite possibly in certain localities of big cities like Chicago, BCG vaccination can be used to advantage on a large scale, and for countries of southeast Asia, it is an excellent procedure. But when the problem reaches the stage of tracking down the last individual infectious cases, in my opinion its use is contra-indicated, except for those specially exposed to infection or likely to be traveling in countries where tuberculosis is common.*

* The position in Cincinnati on June 1, 1963, just before this book went to press was as follows:

By January 31, 1963, every resident of Cincinnati known to have active tuberculosis and a positive sputum was isolated in a hospital. Those who resisted treatment and isolation had been picked up on quarantine orders and placed in the Workhouse Hospital.

By the end of May 1963, the skin testing of the first grade children on a voluntary basis had been completed; 80 per cent of the 11,000 children had been skin tested and 1.6 per cent found to be positive reactors. This test will be compulsory for school entrants commencing September 1963.

Approximately 150 children now attend city clinics or private physicians for prophylactic isoniazid.

Plans are being made to x-ray in 1964 all the residents of high incidence areas over 18 years of age (approximately 60,000). A small scale project along these lines had been attempted in 1950 by the Anti-Tuberculosis League in Cincinnati, but had failed because only 50 per cent of the people came forward to be x-rayed. Very little tuberculosis was found, which probably meant that those who know themselves to have the disease did not come forward to be x-rayed. In 1964, we hope to be more successful in reaching closer to 100 per cent.

REFERENCES

1. COCKBURN, T. A.: The epidemic crisis in East Pakistan 1958. Public Health Rep., 1960, **75**: 26–36.
2. Smallpox 1960–61. W.H.O. Chronicle, **16**: 305.
3. ROGERS, SIR L.: *Smallpox and Climate in India.* Special Reports Series No. 6, Med. Res. Council, H.M. Stationery Office, London, 1926.
4. OLUWOLE, DR. M. O. H. LAGOS: The Smallpox (Shopono) Cult in Nigeria. Précis of a lecture, 1941, Ms.
5. GREENBERG, M.: Complications of vaccination against smallpox. Amer. J. Dis. Child, 1948, **76**: 492–502.
6. DIXON, C. W.: Vaccination against Smallpox. Brit. Med. J., May 5, 1962, pp. 1262–66.
7. DICK, G. W. A.: Prevention of viral infections. Brit. Med. J., Aug. 4, 1962, p. 319.
8. EYLES, D. E., COATNEY, R. G., AND GETZ, M. E.: Vivax-type malaria parasite of Macaques transmissible to man. Science, 1960, **131**: 812–13.
9. CONTACOS, P. G., ELDER, H. A., AND COATNEY, G. R.: Man to man transfer of two strains of *Plasmodium cynomolgi* by mosquito bite. Amer. J. Trop. Med. & Hyg., 1962, **11**: 186–93.
10. W.H.O. Expert Committee on Malaria, W.H.O. Tech. Rep. Ser. *205*, 1961, p. 47.
11. ROMER, A. S.: *The Vertebrate Story.* Univ. of Chicago Press, Chicago, 1959.
12. CARTER, H. R.: *Yellow Fever.* Williams & Wilkins, Baltimore, 1931.
13. GRIFFIN, J. B.: Some Prehistoric Connections between Siberia and America. Science, 1962, **131**: 801–12.
14. WORMINGTON, H. M.: Ancient man in North America. Denver Mus. Nat. Hist., Colorado, 1957.
15. *A Bibliography of Infantile Paralysis 1951.* Ed. FISHBEIN M. and SALMONSEN, E. M. for National Foundation for Infantile Paralysis. J. B. Lippincott Co., Philadelphia, 1951.
16. PORTER, E. R. AND WEHR, R. E.: Oral poliomyelitis vaccine program in Cincinnati. Public Health Rep., 1961, **76**: 369–74.
17. SABIN, A. B.: Community wide use of oral poliovirus vaccine. A.M.A. J. Dis. Child., 1961, **101**: 546–67.
18. COCKBURN, T. A., PORTER, E. R., MACLEOD, K. I. E., LITSEY, J. D., and CROFT, C. C.: Cincinnati's poliomyelitis immunization and surveillance program 1961. Public Health Rep., 1962, **77**: 589–92.
19. HARDIN, G.: The mutual exclusive principle. Science, 1959, **131**: 1292.
20. *Chronicle,* World Health Organization 1960, **14**: 137.
21. GELFAND, H. M., LEBLANC, R., POTASH, L., CLEMMER, D. L., AND FOX, J. P.: The spread of living strains of attenuated poliovirus. Amer. J. Public Health, 1960, **5**: 767.
22. BODIAN, D.: Poliomyelitis, Science, 1955, **122**: 105.
23. COCKBURN, T. A.: Some birds of the Gold Coast with observations on their virus and parasitic infections. Ibis, 1946, **88**: 287–394.
24. MOLLER-CHRISTENSEN, V.: *Bone changes in leprosy.* Munks-gaard, Copenhagen. John Wright and Sons, Bristol, 1961.
25. ALMEIDO, J. O.: Serologic studies in leprosy, W.H.O. Bull., 1962, **26**: 233–40.
25a. McFADZEAN, JAMES A.: Trans. Royal Soc. Trop. Med. Hyg., 1962, **56**: 407–10.
26. YANAGISAWA, KEN: The effect of BCG vaccination upon occurrence of leprosy. Trans. 7th Intern. Cong. Leprosy, pp. 351–56. Jap. Leprosy Foundation, Tokyo, 1958.

27. FROST, W. H.: *The Collected Papers of.* 1946. Ed. Maxy. Commonwealth Fund, New York.
28. Arden House Conference on Tuberculosis, 1959. U.S. Dept. Health, Educ. & Welfare, U.S.P.H.S., Washington, D.C., 1959.
29. HAGAN, W. A.: The control and eradication of animal diseases in the U.S.A. Ann. Rev. Microb., 1958, **12:** 127.

CHAPTER 10

Eradication and the Population Explosion:
The Example of Ceylon*

THE DRAMATIC INCREASE in the rate of growth of the world's population is one of the most serious problems facing the world today. The cause of this is quite clear, the fact being that modern civilization has learned how to prolong the average length of the human life, but not to control within desirable limits the rate of reproduction on a world scale. Various techniques are available for controlling fertilization or ending a pregnancy before a viable fetus has developed, but in many parts of the human race, either because of ignorance or poverty, they cannot be used due to political or religious reasons. The combination of falling death rate and stationary birth rate leads inexorably to what is popularly known as the population explosion (1). The situation is too well publicized to need further exposition here. The fall in the death rate is usually attributed to two main factors—improved food supplies and the application of public health measures, but actual factual documentation of any particular instance is hard to find. The purpose of this chapter is to analyze in some detail one specific incident, the sudden jump in the rate of increase in the population of Ceylon about 1945, and its possible relationship with the application of modern methods of the control and cure of infectious diseases. These became practical for the first time in that country as a result of the ending of World War II. The lesson of the Ceylon experience is that probably the most immediate result of the various eradication programs will be similar jumps in populations in those countries where infectious diseases are the leading agents serving to maintain high death rates. This must not be assumed to indicate that the eradication programs should not be undertaken, but does imply

* The information given in this chapter was collected during the years 1956–58, while I was WHO Advisor in Epidemiology to the government of Ceylon. I am deeply indebted to all my Ceylonese colleagues for the advice and assistance they gave during my stay in their country. All figures, unless otherwise stated, are taken from the files of the Directorate of Health or the Annual Reports of the Director.

233

that hand in hand with such programs should be simultaneous measures to control the rate of reproduction.

The death rate in Ceylon dropped slowly and steadily from 31.0 in 1905 to 22.0 in 1945 at the end of World War II, then suddenly fell to 14.3 in 1946 and continued down to 10.9 in 1953. In parallel with this, the population showed a slow, steady increase since the beginning of the century but suddenly shot up in 1946 (Table 18).

TABLE 18. VITAL STATISTICS CEYLON—1925–55

	Rate of increase	Estimated mid-year population	Birth rate per 1,000 population	Death rate per 1,000 population	Infant mortality rate	Maternal mortality rate
1925		4,846,850	39.9	24.3	172	18.5
1930		5,253,210	39.0	25.1	175	21.4
1935	1.74%	5,608,000	34.4	36.5	263	26.8
1940	1.80%	5,972,000	35.7	20.6	149	16.1
1945	1.81%	6,516,000	36.6	21.9	140	16.5
1946	1.81%	6,719,000	38.2	20.2	141	15.5
1947	2.51%	6,903,000	39.3	14.3	101	10.6
1948	2.74%	7,109,000	40.5	13.2	92	8.3
1949	2.73%	7,321,000	39.8	12.6	87	6.5
1950	2.78%	7,544,000	40.4	12.6	82	5.6
1955	2.69%	8,589,000	37.9	11.0	71	4.1

The rate of increase which was 1.8% during the war rose by nearly 1.0%. There is a close correlation between these figures and the slow improvements in hygiene and medical care up to 1946 and the rapid ones after that time. The two biggest postwar factors were the uses of penicillin and DDT, but the scientific advances were in fact on a wide front and the death rates from many infections were sharply reduced. There has been no great change in birth rate.

Frederiksen (2) has discussed the possible relationship between intensified malaria control in Ceylon in 1947 and the postwar acceleration in the rate of increase in the population. In that country, the first use of DDT on a large scale in 1947 coincided apparently with a sharp rise in the rate of increase, so that the two events were generally considered to be related. Frederiksen concluded that malaria was not responsible for this acceleration. The data presented here supports these findings to some extent; the conclusion is drawn that the drop in the death rate from malaria was only one of many factors, others being the introduction of antibiotics and the application of many new scientific techniques developed during the war.

In 1946, a large number of new discoveries made during World War II became available for general use in Ceylon, so that the mortality rates dropped sharply for many infectious diseases besides malaria. The total drop for all infectious diseases was of the order of magnitude that would be required to explain the increase in population.

Frederiksen, in a later paper (3), holds that there is an association between economic and demographic indices suggesting cause and effecting relationships. He suggests that the health measures were relatively unimportant factors. He even denies that there was any sudden reduction in mortality rates in 1946. However, his own data which he produces in his Figure I to support this contention can easily be interpreted to the contrary. In this Figure, a steady decrease in mortality is apparently indicated by a white bar through the years from 1935 to 1957, with increased mortality for the war years. A better interpretation for this data would be a horizontal bar for the years 1935 to 1946, indicating no change in the mortality rates during that period, a sharp drop in 1946, and a sloping one for the subsequent years showing a continuous reduction in the mortality rates in that time.

Medical Care in Ceylon

There are two forms of medical care in Ceylon (Figure 19), the so-called Western medicine and the indigenous type or Ayurvedic medicine. Ayurvedic medicine has a long history in the country, dating back to prehistoric times, and the main tenents were compiled by teachers such as Susruta as long ago as 3,000 years. Many of the treatments and dietary regimes in use then were as advanced as those employed today in Western medicine so that, for example, the patient suffering from infectious hepatitis 3,000 years ago would have received basically the same treatment as one in a hospital in England or the United States today. Many of the drug preparations used are highly potent and one of these, Rauwolfia, has recently been introduced to the Western world for use in high blood pressure and as a tranquilizer.

Before World War II, Ayurvedic physicians competed successfully with practitioners of Western medicine in many fields. Up to that time, the drugs available that had specific therapeutic value for common ailments could have been counted on the fingers of both hands, and most of these used by Western physicians could usually be obtained also by Ayurvedic physicians. The Ayurvedic physicians were present in all areas, while their Western counterparts congregated in the cities, and also the former charged a good deal less for their services. For every Western physician in practice there must have been about ten Ayurvedic ones. In 1951, Ayurvedic physicians were invited to apply for registration and 12,957 application forms were requested. In 1955, there were 7,400 registered

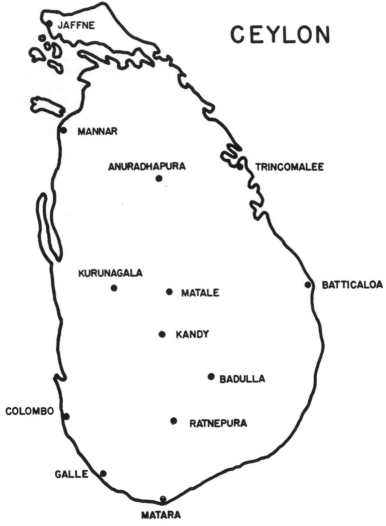

Figure 19. Map of Ceylon.

Ayurvedic physicians as well as an unknown number practicing without registration. The numbers of Western practitioners are given in Table 19. It is obvious that the greater mass of illness, excluding that requiring surgery, must have been treated by the Ayurvedic practitioners.

TABLE 19. WESTERN PHYSICIANS

	Apothecaries	Gov't. physicians	Private practice
1940	?	234	693
1946	551	561	486
1955	990	838	929

With the end of World War II, this position changed dramatically. Penicillin and a number of other "wonder" drugs suddenly flooded the market. These drugs were highly potent, and the ordinary citizen

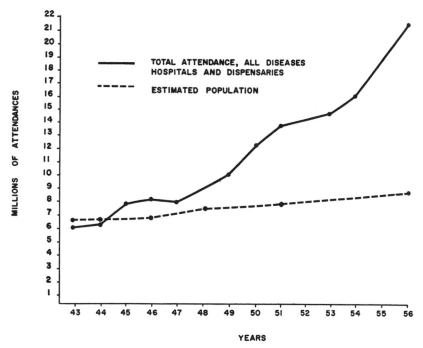

Figure 20. Morbidity and Population—Ceylon, 1943–56.

who was ill was quick to appreciate the fact that usually they relieved his suffering and cured his illness.

The first result of this was a marked rise in the numbers of people attending the Western type hospitals and dispensaries, most of them demanding or expecting inoculations of antibiotics. This rise is illustrated in Figure 20, where it will be seen that the rate of increase of attendance was greatly in excess of the corresponding rise in population. The second result was the demand by the Ayurvedic physicians for training in antibiotics, although their philosophy was incompatible with the germ theory of disease that had produced these antibiotics.* The increased competition led to the formation of a College of Ayurvedic Physicians in 1956, the attempts to license the various practitioners, and efforts to raise the standards of Ayurvedic practice. Considerable pressure was exerted on the government to provide training in the use of antibiotics for Ayurvedic physicians.†

The increased demand for medical services led in turn to their provision on an increasing scale. Tables 19 and 20 show the extent of this with regard to hospitals, hospital beds, dispensaries, number of physicians, and money spent. The increase in antibiotics bought for general use is also indicated by the samples given in Table 21, the increase applying to all the antibiotics, including sulfa drugs.

* On several occasions, the Minister of Health, Mrs. Wimala Wijewardene, asked me to teach the Ayurvedic physicians to use antibiotics. Under the conditions prevailing at this time, this was impossible. However, some Ayurvedic physicians were already using penicillin and sulfa drugs, and it is only a matter of time before this practice becomes general. Presumably they will become better organized and trained, so that eventually their practices will approximate those of Western physicians. The exchange of knowledge need not be one way. They have much to teach the Western world, especially with regard to drugs as well as in the approach to the patient. In their philosophy, the patient is an individual, and not merely a collection of organs as regarded so frequently in hospitals of the U.S. today. The valuable preparation, Rauwolfia, and its derivative, Reserpine, came within the past two decades from a study of the Ayurvedic pharmacopoeia.

† The depth of the feeling of the Ayurvedic physicians with regard to Western medicine and especially antibiotics can be measured by the fact that it was a major factor in the assassination of Ceylon's Prime Minister, Mr. Bandaranaike. Of the six people arrested, one was the Minister of Health, who strongly supported the training of Ayurvedic physicians in the use of antibiotics, another was a lecturer at the College of Ayurvedic Medicine, while the assassin was a Buddhist monk and herbalist.

"In Colombo last week, a Buddhist monk and herbalist named Talduwe Somarama mounted a prison scaffold and was hanged. Somarama's crime: the 1959 assassination of Ceylon's Prime Minister Solomon W. R. D. Bandaranaike. In a confession he later retracted, Somarama said he committed the deed because the Prime Minister favored Western medical techniques over Oriental herb medicine. Prison officials reported that 24 hours before he was hanged, Somarama had himself baptized a Christian so that he could ask God for the forgiveness of sin that cannot be found in the Buddhist religion." *Time,* July 13, 1962, p. 36.

These drugs are not used so lavishly in Ceylon as in the U.S., so that more value per tablet is obtained in the former.

In 1945, the population was increasing at the rate of 1.8 per cent and this rate had not changed markedly for some years. For an extra

TABLE 20. MEDICAL FACILITIES

	Hospitals	Hospital beds	Central dispensaries	Rupees per capita
1940	129	11,425	268	2.22
1946	189	16,787	240	4.27
1956	381	25,482	283	10.90

increase of about 0.1 per cent with the birth rate remaining stationary, about 1,000 people per million population would have to survive who normally would be expected to die. With a population of 6.5 million, such an increase would need 6,500 additional survivors.

TABLE 21. ANTIBIOTICS FOR GENERAL ISSUE GOVERNMENT MEDICAL STORES

	Penicillin millions of units	Chloromycetin tablets	P.A.S. millions of tablets
1945	—	—	—
1952–53	372.2	296,178	13.0
1955–56	1217.4	615,271	56.6

By 1956, the rate of increase in the population of 8.8 million had risen by almost 0.9 per cent over the 1945 level, requiring about 80,000 people per year to survive who would have died had the 1945 death rates still prevailed.

TABLE 22. REPORTED DEATHS FROM CERTAIN INFECTIOUS DISEASES *

	Malaria	Typhoid	Ankylostomiasis	Pulmonary T.B.	Dysentery & enteritis	Pneumonia
1940	9,169	988	1,606	3,299	6,766	9,084
1945	8,539	1,471	1,819	3,268	7,325	9,321
1950	1,903	671	933	3,694	3,458	7,588
1956	16	201	201	853	2,030	2,221

* The reliability of these data is discussed in the text. It must be emphasized that Ceylonese physicians are usually graduates of the Medical College at Colombo which is one of the best in South East Asia. All professors and consultants have graduate degrees, most of these being from British Universities. The standards of diagnosis and laboratory facilities provided in the rural areas are probably comparable to those in the U.S. a few decades ago, while those in Colombo are probably equal to that in small towns in the U.S. at the present time. The actual reporting of what is diagnosed is incomparably better than in the U.S.

The numbers of deaths from the major killing infections in certain selected years are given in Table 22. This is based largely on data from government hospitals. It will be seen that the numbers reported for each infection have declined sharply, although not only has the population sharply increased but also the percentage of people using the hospitals as described earlier. In interpreting these figures, the fact must be remembered that Ayurvedic physicians cannot report causes of death since their concept of illness differs markedly from that of Western physicians, and secondly, that hospital data reflects chiefly the conditions in towns where there are hospitals and not the rural places that are far from hospitals. However, most probably only few deaths fail to be reported even though the nature of the fatal illness may be obscure. Most Ayurvedic physicians hasten to unburden themselves of patients whose conditions seem likely to terminate in death. In 1956, total deaths reported were 88,971 and of these 23,193, or about 25 per cent, occurred in government hospitals. Allowing for the bias in the figures as indicated, it appears that a crude estimate of the total deaths for easily diagnosed specific infections could be obtained by multiplying the reported hospital figures by a factor of about four.

The difference in the total numbers of deaths from killing infections in Table 22 for 1945 and 1956 is 27,362; when this is multiplied by the factor of 4.0 to correct for the underreporting and allowance is made for the differences in the population figures for the two years, it will be clear that the increase in population can be accounted for almost entirely by these six categories of infectious diseases. Any deficiencies can be made up by including other infectious diseases that are not so numerous, but which have also responded well to modern preventive or medical measures. Included in this group are puerperal sepsis, the rural form of filariasis but not the urban kind, diphtheria, treponemal infections, leprosy, amebiasis, etc.

More detailed analyses of the various killing infections are now given, preceded by a brief account of pyrexias of unknown origin.

Pyrexias of Unknown Origin—"Malaria" and "Influenza"

In Ceylon at the beginning of the present century, both the facilities for diagnosis as well as the status of scientific knowledge were very inadequate, so that precise information is lacking as to the relative importance of various infections. Obvious diseases such as smallpox, plague, cholera, and often malaria and typhoid would be recognized, but a large mass of disease could not be differentiated. Febrile illnesses were therefore classified according to their characteristics, such as simple continued fever, relapsing fever, undulant fever, or if the elevation of temperature lasted more than seven days, it was often called typhoid fever. Usually these terms did not mean the same as is meant today, so that undulant fever was not necessarily brucellosis but merely a fever that undulated. The term "malaria" included a lot of illnesses that were not plasmodial.

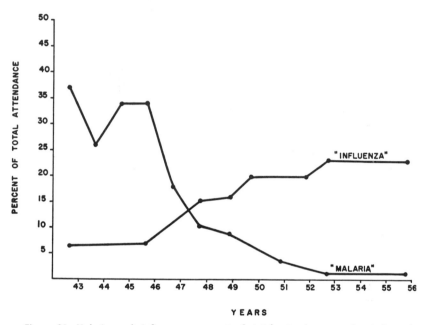

Figure 21. Malaria and Influenza per cent of total attendance at hospitals and dispensaries in Ceylon, 1943–56.

Today "influenza" is the commonest diagnosis made in hospitals and dispensaries, forming about 23 per cent of the total reported and 50 per cent of the infectious diseases. It does not refer to infection with influenza virus, but is a term employed for all the mass of undiagnosable short term pyrexias so frequently seen in the country. At a meeting of the Medical Research Group in Colombo in 1956, Dr. A. Amarasinha pointed out that the term had come into general use quite recently, in fact about 1947–48. This was a time when the diagnosis of malaria as a catch-all for undiagnosable fevers was becoming increasingly unpopular owing to the activities of the

TABLE 23. "INFLUENZA" IN COLUMBO: PAIRED SERA FROM TYPICAL PATIENTS TESTED AGAINST SIX ARBOR VIRUSES

Name	Age	Date of collection	Complement fixation						Hemagglutination inhibition				
			JBE	MVE	TN	E101	DNI	TR	JBE	MVE	TN	E101	TR
M. I. Haladeen	37	6.7.56	4	8	4	<4	16	32	4	5	4	5	5
M. I. Haladeen	37	26.7.56	64	64	32	8	512	512	9	>10	9	>10	>10
K. P. Karunawathie	33	13.7.56	<4	<4	<4	<4	<4	4	3	3	2	4	4
K. P. Karunawathie	33	3.8.56	8	8	16	8	16	16	4	4	3	4	5
E. K. E. Jinadasa	25	16.7.56	<4	<4	<4	<4	<4	<4	0	0	0	0	0
E. K. E. Jinadasa	25	6.8.56	128	128	16	8	16	128	8	8	7	7	7
L. B. Dharmasena	22	12.7.56	<4	<4	<4	<4	<4	<4	0	0	0	0	1
L. B. Dharmasena	22	28.7.56	64	128	128	64	512	512	9	9	8	8	10
K. P. Karunapathe	25	7.8.56	<4	<4	<4	<4	<4	<4	0	0	0	0	0
K. P. Karunapathe	25	29.8.56	8	8	8	<4	64	64	10	10	9	10	10
M. D. Piyasena	13	28.8.56	<4	<4	<4	<4	<4	<4	2	2	0	2	4
M. D. Piyasena	13	17.9.56	256	256	128	32	128	256	10	10	8	10	10

officers of the Anti-Malaria Campaign. As the malaria began to disappear from the island, reports of cases received increasing attention and were followed by requests for blood smears. As a result, another name had to be given to these non-malarial pyrexias and apparently the one most used was that of "influenza."

This point is illustrated in Figure 21, where it will be seen that before 1947 about 25 to 35 per cent of the total attendance for all illnesses was said to be malaria, but that after 1947 when malaria disappeared, a new feature arose in that a previously minor amount of illness called "influenza," forming about 8 per cent of the total, suddenly jumped to prominence and remained steady at 23 per cent of the total. The likelihood of a new disease suddenly appearing in this fashion is rather small, so that the most probable explanation is that all the time about 23 per cent of the total illness had been this non-malarial pyrexia. About 8 per cent had been called "influenza" and the remaining 15 per cent "malaria." The removal of the true malaria unmasked the non-malarial infections previously given that name and led to the increased reporting of "influenza" (Figure 21).

A study of cases of typical "influenza" was made as a co-operative effort by many members of the Medical Research Group in 1957. It was finally shown that probably much of it was due to infections by arbor viruses. Specimens of sera were collected in the acute and convalescent phases of the illnesses by Drs. I. Vaithianathan and A. Viswaratnam, Medical College, Colombo, and tested by Dr. Telford Work at Poona, India. Rising titers against a number of arbor viruses were demonstrated. Typical examples are given in Table 23. A survey of 400 sera collected by the Blood Bank showed a high percentage to have antibodies against these viruses.

Malaria

Malaria in Ceylon has been described in some detail by Frederiksen and will therefore receive no special analysis in this paper.

Tuberculosis

Tuberculosis control on a large scale had not been attempted in Ceylon until the early forties, any efforts before that time being limited to treatment of cases. In 1941, efforts at prevention were first contemplated and a batch of medical officers sent for training.

A committee was set up and its recommendations published as a Sessional Paper in 1945 (S.P. 111–1945). A superintendent of the Tuberculosis Campaign was appointed in 1946, and after that the anti-tuberculosis movement developed rapidly. With the assistance of WHO and UNICEF, a BCG campaign was organized in 1949. Several visiting experts gave advice and the Australian government made a gift of three million rupees for the campaign. Modern clinics with facilities for quick and rapid diagnosis were opened up at Galle, Ratnapura, Kandy, Kurunegala, Jaffne and Anuradhapura.

The campaigns received considerable impetus from all these activities, so that by 1954 there were seven BCG teams in action in the field, and in the six year program nearly a million people had been vaccinated. In 1956, a survey estimated cases of unhealed pathology to be about 63,000. Antibiotics active against the tubercle bacillus became available in Ceylon soon after World War II, and by the 1950's large quantities were being imported. As a result, the domiciliary treatment of this disease was becoming practical.

The death rate from pulmonary tuberculosis for several years is given in Table 22. Allowing for the fact that all the increased activity would have resulted in a much greater rate of case finding, the figures still indicate that not much progress in the reduction of mortality occurred before 1949, but from that year to 1956, the number of deaths dropped sharply.

Smallpox, Cholera, Plague

Prior to 1899, much disease had been imported from India, being carried by laborers immigrating to the tea and rubber estates. There had been unrestricted immigration of this kind through the Pamban-Mannar route known as the "North Route." From Mannar the men marched to Matale a distance of 148 miles, halting at many places en route and leaving behind a trail of dirt and infection. In 1899, alarmed at epidemics of plague, cholera, and smallpox in India, the Ceylon government set up an advisory committee to advise on the prevention of introduction of infectious diseases from abroad. The success of the measures of quarantine recommended by this Committee and enforced over subsequent years can be seen in Table 24.

By the 1930's, smallpox and cholera had been eliminated as indigenous infections, and only occurred in small outbreaks when brought in from India. During the war years, this rigid quarantine broke down to some degree and there was an upsurge in these diseases.

Plague had been imported from India, but was confined to a few localized areas and died out in 1937.

In the 1950's, plague, cholera, and smallpox were absent from Ceylon except when an occasional case slipped through the quarantine, usually as a result of illegal immigration from India. In 1957, a small outbreak of 24 cases of smallpox resulted from a small boy developing the modified disease six days after arriving in the country; he had been vaccinated in India and developed a few vesicles that were pronounced to be chickenpox by three competent and experi-

TABLE 24. ANNUAL AVERAGE OF CASES

	Smallpox	Cholera
1871–80	—	3,675
1881–90	1,162	386
1891–00	309	612
1901–10	351	171
1911–20	175	110
1921–30	83	42
1931–40	65	9
1941–50	156	24

enced physicians. In 1956, there were about 14 cases of a cholera-like disease in the Jaffna area that were probably also due to illegal immigration.

Roundworm and Hookworm

The incidence of hookworm and roundworm forms a good index of sanitary conditions. A seminar on this subject was held in Colombo by the Medical Research Group on June 26, 1957, when all those with long experience in Ceylon agreed that both the severity of infection and the numbers of persons parasitized has been reduced in the past few decades. The data produced at this meeting is summarized in Tables 25 and 26. No early figures could be found for roundworm incidence. There is no way of comparing the number of worms per person over these decades, but the general concensus of the meeting was that the patients with marked clinical symptoms such as gross anemia in hookworm and intestinal obstruction in roundworm are rarities now, whereas 20 years earlier they had been everyday events in all large outpatient clinics. The data available and the clinical impressions of the physicians support the idea that there has been a slow but steady improvement of sanitary conditions over the years.

Infestation with parasites like these is not usually regarded as an important direct cause of death. However, the massive and general prevalence of these worms in Ceylon must be an important contributing factor to a general lowering of the public health and wel-

TABLE 25. HOOKWORM SURVEYS

Location	Source of data	Year	Number examined	Number infected	Percentage infected
All provinces	Rockefeller Foundation	1916 1924–25	7,645 32,507	7,358 29,433	96.2% 90.5%
All provinces	Ankylostomiasis Campaign	1933	—	—	81.4%
	Directorate of Health Services	1937	—	—	74.1%
Kurunegala (small children)	Environmental sanitation project	1956	291	136	46.7%

TABLE 26. ROUNDWORM SURVEYS

Location	Source of data	Year	Number examined	Number infected	Percentage infected
All provinces	Ankylostomiasis Campaign	1950–55	2,599	1,745	67%
Kurunegala (children)	Environmental sanitation project	1956	291	221	75.8%
Lady Ridgeway Hospital (children)	Department of Pediatrics	1950–54	5,860	2,267	38.7%

fare. It must be a significant indirect cause toward a high death rate in early life. Without doubt, there have been substantial improvements in this situation with past decades, and these have accelerated since the war with the provision of new anti-helminthics and the campaigns of the government to provide more and better latrines. This progress is reflected in the figures of deaths from ankylostomiasis in Table 25. Early figures are not available for roundworm infestation incidence.

Typhoid

Typhoid is obviously very common in Ceylon, but accurate statistics are difficult to find since without adequate laboratory services the diagnosis can be impossible.* In 1956–57, in collaboration with the Medical Research Institute, a study was begun to attempt an estimate of the amount of typhoid in the country. This consisted of an analysis of the records in the Directorate of Health, the investigation of epidemics, and a concentrated field study in the town of Panadura. Panadura, with a population of about 21,000, is about 14 miles from Colombo; in 1956, there were 97 cases of typhoid diagnosed in the hospital and of these 27 were residents of the town. There had also been 28 cases of simple continued fever reported from the town, and cross-checking with the Institute revealed that serologically most of these were typhoid cases that had not been reported as such. Many cases were seen that were labeled "influenza," while others were treated by the Ayurvedic practitioners and so would not be recognized as typhoid. (The Singhalese name for typhoid is "Una sunni pathe" meaning fever affecting the brain.) The conclusion was drawn that only about one case in ten is seen by a Western physician, diagnosed correctly, and finally reported to the Directorate of Health. This level of reporting to a health authority is equivalent to that of syphilis in the United States.

The findings in Panadura were confirmed during an epidemic in 1957 in Kurunagala that was investigated in some detail. About one case in ten had been reported.

The conclusion drawn was that about 20,000 to 40,000 cases of typhoid occur in Ceylon every year. The importance of this to the population figures is that since World War II a potent antibiotic in the form of chloromycetin has been available, and this has cut down the death rate sharply. As can be seen from Table 21, the import of this drug has risen considerably in recent years, and without doubt, many people are living today in Ceylon because of this drug who would have died without it. The reduction in deaths from typhoid from 1945 to 1956 as shown in Table 22 is obviously an underestimate.

---

* The clinical description of the disease given in Western textbooks is not that commonly seen in Ceylon. Most frequently the only feature is a pyrexia, often with constipation. The traditional Singhalese name "fever affecting the brain" is very accurate.

Discussion

Data have been presented that clearly illustrate three points: First, the rate of increase of population in Ceylon jumped markedly immediately after World War II terminated, secondly, this increase can be explained by the decrease in the deaths caused by the main groups of infectious diseases, and thirdly, this reduction was caused by the application of new methods of prevention and treatment of infectious diseases. The cost per capita of the medical services that achieved this result rose from Rs. 4.27 in 1946 to Rs. 10.90 in 1956, which is a comparatively modest rise when compared to the total economy of the country and is even smaller when allowance is made for inflation.

Why did the increase occur when it did and why have other neighboring countries like East Pakistan failed to react in the same way? The answer to the first question must be that before 1946 all new drugs and equipments were in very short supply so that the increase could not have happened earlier, but that immediately when the war ended Ceylon was in an excellent position to obtain and utilize these commodities. The country emerged undamaged and prosperous from the war and with its products of tea, rubber, and copra in great demand. It has an ideal position on the sea routes of the world. It has one of the best medical services in southeast Asia.

East Pakistan, on the contrary, is a poor country that was near the front line of the fighting. It had an appalling famine in 1943 that killed several million people. At the Partition of India in 1947, it lost not only its access to Calcutta, the main port of the area, but also most of its doctors. They were Hindu and fled to India. Communications are very bad since the land is largely flooded every year for three or four months and roads become largely non-existent. Accurate statistics are hard to get, but the rate of increase is probably still about 1.8 as was that of Ceylon before 1945.

However, improvements are in progress: New roads and ports are being built, pure water for every village is being supplied, new medical schools are beginning to pour out many hundreds of doctors every year, and plans are in preparation for the eradication of diseases such as smallpox and malaria. I have estimated elsewhere (4) that if all these plans are put into effect successfully, that in ten years' time, the rate of increase in East Pakistan will rise by the same degree as did that in Ceylon. In fact if an extra four or five rupees per annum per head were made available in most countries in south-east Asia, and the money was spent on preventive medicine instead of hospitals, the rate of increase of population in the whole of this area could be raised rapidly to close to 3.0 per cent per annum.

Rates of population increases of this magnitude pose many problems. Since the rate of increase of productivity of this part of the world is unlikely for some time to exceed 2.0 per cent, there is every prospect of the welfare of the people going backward instead of forward. Birth control is not the answer at present; for the next decade or two its effect will be scarcely comparable with the opposing measures of preventive medicine. Some major scientific breakthrough in this field will be necessary before a deliberate major reduction of the birth rate will be practical. Nor can the benefits of public health and medical care be denied to the people of any country, for as the example of Ceylon shows (Figure 21) when the people realize that scientific treatments can alleviate their sufferings, they demand these and the government has to supply them. No leader of a people would dare tell his countrymen that every year tens of thousands of them must die horrible deaths from leprosy, tuberculosis, etc., just because the productivity cannot increase fast enough.

The world population explosion is one of the greatest problems of this era, equal in size to that of nuclear warfare. It is becoming both a major nightmare for the statesman and a conflict of conscience for the individual. It is not so much a religious matter over the question of birth control—for the techniques for controlling population in this fashion that are presently available are simply not practical in underdeveloped countries—but one of making progress in material prosperity at the cost of preventible human suffering and death. Infectious disease is obviously one of the main factors limiting population's size, and indeed may be the controlling factor in areas where the food supplies are above the critical minimum. The various infections can usually be eliminated at very small cost, but the people who have been thus saved from dying will need food, clothing, homes, and work, and these may not be available if there are too many of them. In many parts of the world today it is argued "why should a baby be saved from some infection soon after birth only to die of hunger ten years later?" This kind of question determines the low priorities given to health programs in many countries and is reflected in much of the thinking of those allocating U.S. funds for assistance to foreign countries. The counter-argument is that we cannot let die millions of people who could be saved at little expense; that progress at this price is too expensive. This is truly one of the great dilemmas of our time.

REFERENCES

1. DORN, H. F.: 1962. World population growth. Science, 1962, **135:** 283–90.
2. FREDERIKSEN, H.: Malaria control and population pressure in Ceylon, Public Health Rep., 1960, **75:** 865–68.
3. FREDERIKSEN, H.: Determinants and consequences of mortality trends in Ceylon. Public Health Rep., 1962, **76:** 659–64.
4. COCKBURN, T. A.: Infectious Disease and the Population of East Pakistan. Seminar on Population Growth and Economic Development. Institute of Development Economics Karachi, 1959, pp. 297–302.

Index